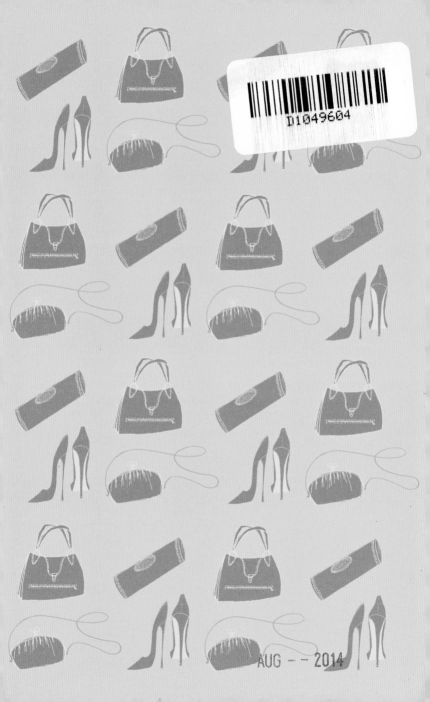

How to be
a Lady

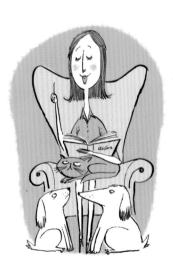

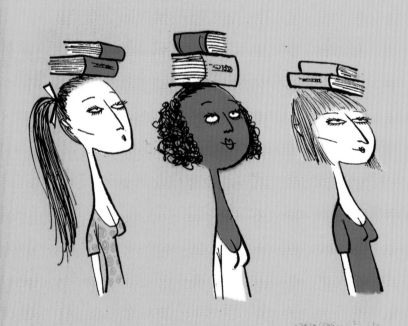

How to be
a Lady

Expert advice on manners
for aspiring sophisticates

Alexandra Parsons
Illustrations by Lord Dunsby

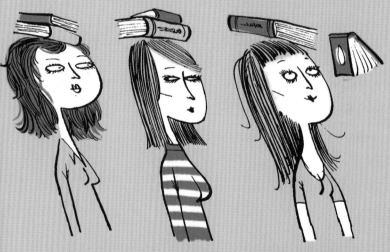

CICO BOOKS
LONDON NEW YORK

Published in 2014 by CICO Books
An imprint of Ryland Peters & Small Ltd
20–21 Jockey's Fields   519 Broadway, 5th Floor
London WC1R 4BW   New York, NY 10012

www.rylandpeters.com

10 9 8 7 6 5 4 3 2 1

Text © Alexandra Parsons 2014
Design and photography © CICO Books 2014

A CIP catalog record for this book is available from the
Library of Congress and the British Library.

ISBN: 978 1 78249 115 6

Printed in China

Editor: Rosanna Lewis
Designer: Jerry Goldie
Illustrator: Steve Millington aka Lord Dunsby

For digital editions, visit www.cicobooks.com/apps.php

Contents

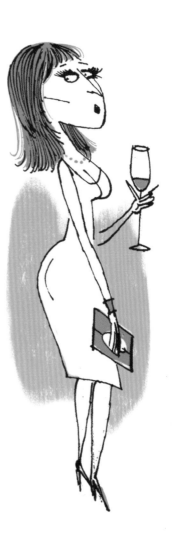

Introduction

—◆—

The great secret... is not having bad manners or good manners or any other particular sort of manners, but having the same manner for all human souls.

George Bernard Shaw, *Pygmalion* (1912)

Why bother with the social graces? The fact is that good manners, a pleasant disposition and an air of confidence are valuable assets in easing a graceful path through life, and you get the best out of people when they get the best of you. Good manners aren't formulas to learn, they are about being nice, kind and considerate, but it does also help if you look pleasantly clean and unthreatening, speak clearly and stand up straight.

But it's not actually enough to be the thoughtful, well-spoken sort of person. A lady needs to be the type of party guest who does not cut the nose off the cheese, is capable of opening an oyster and knows the correct way to introduce a hip-hop artist to a boy scout. Although all these skills are vital, it's perhaps even more vital not to be bland or boring. Ladies must have character and wit and go about life with panache.

Don't take this book too seriously... I certainly didn't... but check it out – you may find some good sense and useful tips to help you define yourself as a couth (taking this to be the opposite of uncouth) individual with a sense of fun and a knack for putting everyone at ease.

My mother had all the attributes of ladylike-ness, including the eccentric bits, so it is to her memory I dedicate this book. As a child I was not always the epitome of couth, being naturally a little scruffy round the edges, and I can still hear her withering tones of disappointment: "Alexandra, you just WANT to be a rough girl!" Well, the rough girl came good, and so can you.

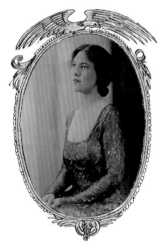

Margaret Elizabeth Towle (neé Ginders)

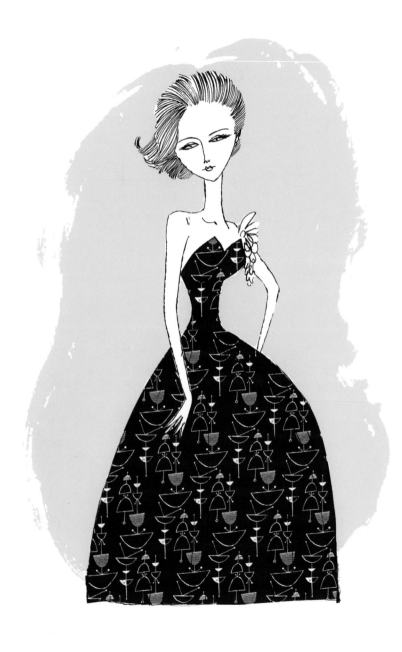

Chapter 1

How to Look
Like a Lady

———◆———

*As to matters of dress,
I would recommend one never
to be first in the fashion
nor the last out of it.*

John Wesley (1703–1791),
English evangelist and founder of Methodism.
Right on, John.

Getting The Hang
of Getting Dressed

It's dead obvious, really. A lady will dress appropriately for her size and age, and the occasion. She will not dress to outrage or stand out from the crowd. She will look just lovely: poised, effortless and unruffled. A lady will edit her wardrobe, choosing a select few well-cut, flattering outfits, suitable for her figure, in proper fabrics such as linen, cotton, wool and silk, leaving 100% polyester numbers on the hanger, in the shop. Her clothes will be bandbox fresh and appropriate for the time of day. This level of cool is not easy to achieve as it requires dedication to the washing machine, the dry-cleaner, the iron and the mending box, and being bothered to fold clothes tidily and hang things up. It also requires the ability to get in touch with one's internal trash-ometer.

Nothing screams 'TRASH!' quite so loudly as a hefty woman bulging out of a small frock. The generously endowed of any age should avoid short, tight, low-cut outfits. Most extreme fashions are not considered ladylike because they scream for attention, and ladies don't do that. If you are young, slender and beautiful, you can get away with a great deal, but there is a world of difference between taut, healthy and stunning and turning out like a junior-league, surgically enhanced celeb strutting her assets in buttock-

> **A tip:** Don't be obsessed by the size on the label. Buy what fits you properly, and if you're feeling sensitive, just cut out the offending tag and be the size you want to be. It will make you feel better and stop skinnier 'friends' riffling through your wardrobe for a good sneer.

revealing shorts and ripped tights. A finely tuned trash-ometer will help you to tell the difference.

A Shortlist of Unladylike Items:

* Tight white jeans

* Any cheap white skirts or trousers you can see through

* Cheap, thin, transparent tops, unless you have the body of a goddess

* Thigh-high boots

* Fake-leather anything

There will be times, however, when you need to dress to stand out from the crowd. For this you need a lot of self-assurance and something stunningly out-of-the-ordinary, such as a vintage or ethnic garment or an outrageous hat. Avoid anything gaudy, tacky or so high-fashion that it makes you look enslaved.

Personal Grooming

If you are very, very, very posh, you may be able to get away with unshaven armpits, rank breath and hair like a rat's nest, but only because people lose their perspective around the peaks of privilege, protecting the inbred and spoilt with the cloak of eccentricity. Eccentrics are rarely contented people, and they don't often get invited to the same place twice. So: wash, take good care of your nails and feet, moisturise your neck and find a hairstyle that suits you and looks kempt. Why? Because a lady will always make herself pleasant to be around.

If your teeth are awful, get them fixed so that they look natural but white-ish and straight-ish, and don't get sucked in by a Teeth-capping Whitening Makeover. Totally even, sparkling teeth look fake and terribly unladylike. The same goes for large silicone breasts. Don't use an overpowering scent, and don't use overpowering amounts of any scent. If you wear the same perfume all

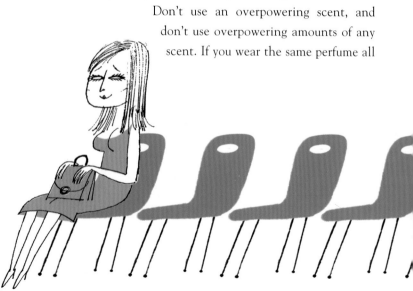

day every day, you will become immune to it and end up using toxic amounts, so rotate different fragrances and be aware of the scents of body lotions and face creams you may be adding to the mix. Heavy, musky perfumes are to be avoided: no lady should smell like a cat on heat.

Perfume comes in several strengths, and it goes without saying that the most expensive is the strongest:

* Perfume (use just a hint)

* Eau de parfum (a dab will do)

* Eau de toilette (a couple of quick bursts)

* Eau de cologne (splash it about a bit)

{ **A tip:** Spray perfume into the air in front of you and walk into the cloud. Enough will settle to make you smell alluring. }

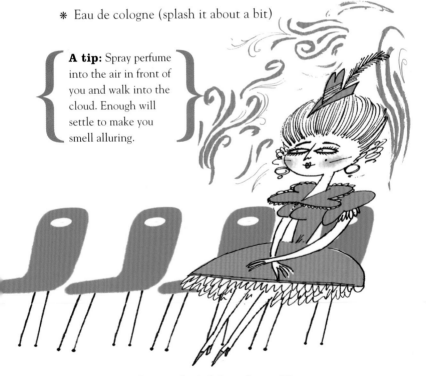

> *Very stout persons should never wear white. It has the effect of adding to the bulk of the figure.*
>
> Sound advice from
> **Routledge's Manual of Etiquette**,
> first published in the late nineteenth century.

Underwear

This should be fit for purpose and co-ordinated with the colour of your outfit. So, no black knickers under white trousers or brilliant white bras advertising themselves underneath slinky black tops. Nude colours are a good option. Too much lace is not good, because it is hard for clothes to fit well over clumps of crispy froth. If white underwear goes grey or blue in the wash, throw it out; those lingerie whiteners never really work. (Note to self: get on the case.) Thongs? I don't think so. If you were to get run over by the proverbial bus, you'd be comforted to know the ambulance crew and the emergency-room team would immediately know how ladylike you are (were) from your clean, well-fitting

{ **A thought to ponder:** The word 'lingerie' comes from the French *lin*, meaning linen; it later referred to all washable items, as in *laver le linge* meaning DO THE WASHING … }

underwear. Cute is fine for the very, very young, but the lady will avoid graphic sexual messages and/or stupid jokes writ large upon her bottom. Tights aren't very sexy, but they are wonderfully functional and it's nice to know that the more expensive, finer deniers are the least likely to snag and run. A lady with foresight will keep a spare pair of tights in her bag, and no lady will ever wear pop socks with skirts.

Party Wear

This brings up the cleavage/leg question. The traditional answer is 'one or the other', as revealing both looks trashy.

If you have religious qualms with legs and arms, there are plenty of stylish, modest party dresses to choose from that do not shout 'LOOK AT ME, I AM THE HOLIEST PERSON IN THE ROOM', which is in itself attention-grabbing and therefore as deeply unladylike as turning up half-naked.

Ladies who wish to dress alluringly for a party do so with good undergarments, several hours of preparation and the help of a full-length mirror.

Ladies who wish to dress alluringly for a party do so with good undergarments, several hours of preparation and the help of a full-length mirror.

Ladies for whom the social round is absolutely not a big deal and nothing to get fussed about can race in from the hunting field or vegetable patch with minutes to spare, kick off their rubber Wellington boots (Hunter's, of course), scrub their faces with a flannel, brush the hay out of their hair, cram on a tiara and dive into a ball gown. But you have to have panache to get away with that (a stately home and a title would also help).

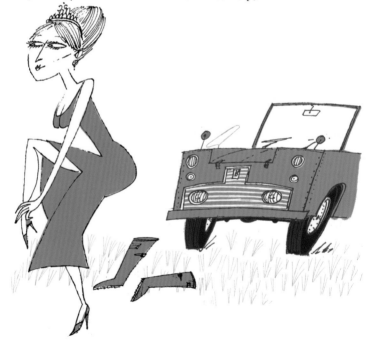

Formal Occasions

Some invitations stipulate a dress code. This is so that everyone is dressed to the same level and no one feels uncomfortably over- or underdressed – it's nothing to get all revolutionary about. Here are the codes, just so you don't have to go and look them up anywhere else. I don't know how significant it is that dress codes are addressed to men. Maybe this is something to get revolutionary about?

White tie signifies a very rare, extremely formal event requiring proper ball gowns, top hats, tiaras and gloves and stuff. If you mix in that kind of circle, what are you doing reading this book?

Black tie indicates smart evening wear. For women this means a cocktail dress, long or short but not too short, and any colour you like, including black.

Morning dress is often used for weddings or a race meeting where you might bump into a member of the royal family. It means formal day wear: a smart suit or knee-length dress and probably a hat.

Evening wear means smart and eveningy (but not as uptight as black tie).

Smart casual means exactly what it says. Clean and comfortable: no jeans, no sportswear.

Weddings And Funerals

Wedding guests should not wear white, upstage the bride, or get tragically drunk.

For a funeral, wear dark colours in moderation; there's no need to go over the top with the black. Dramas can and do occur at funerals, so if you are in the sad position of burying a husband or lover, it's best to look as stunning as you possibly can under the circumstances (think veil, dark glasses and a snappy hat), just in case a second family or long-term mistress slips into the back pew.

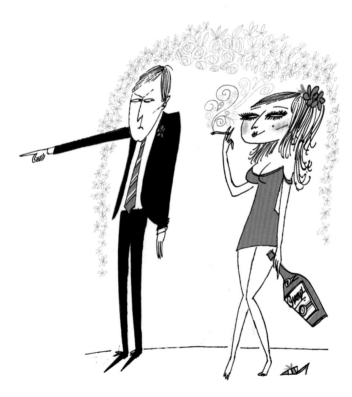

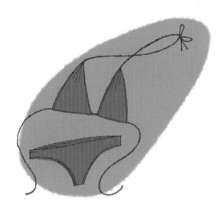

Beachwear

Indulge in a pedicure and a leg and bikini-line wax. Buy swimwear that fits and flatters, and invest in a decent beach towel – a threadbare rag is a horrible sight. A good floaty cover-up is essential for visiting beach bars, as are some decent flat sandals (tottering about in the sand in high heels is not a good look). Ladies do not get sunburned; they stay in the shade, wear sun-hats and maintain their cool. If they wear jewellery to the beach it will be an understated rope of coral or seashells. No bling.

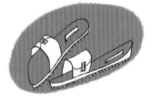

A girl should be two things: classy and fabulous.

Coco Chanel (1883–1971),
designer and populariser of the suntan.

Hats

Lovely big hats top off formal daywear, and – as long as you can keep them on – they solve all hairstyle dilemmas at the stab of a hatpin. Big hats look good on tall women with slim-fitting suits or dresses. A big hat, full skirt and baggy top equals fashion disaster and, if the wind gets up, probably a hazard to light aircraft. Social kissing in big hats is something to practise. Imagine two ladies in cartwheels of hats approaching each other for a 'mwah mwah'. It's best to approach with your head slightly tilted one way or another, so the approaching hat picks up the hint and tilts her head the other way.

Big hats, little hats, witty hats, fascinators, veils and clip-on sprouts of feathers all have their place in the hat pantheon,

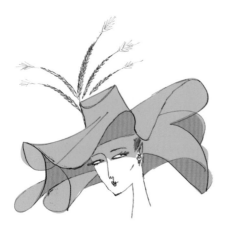

and the secret of looking ladylike with a hat on is a question of balance. Overwrought hair and hats do not mix well. Look at the outfit as a whole in a full-length mirror. Be mindful of colour co-ordination and silhouette, and bear in mind hat practicalities: will you have to slip through doors sideways; will the people sitting in the row behind you have to use periscopes to see?

Gloves

Once upon a time, no lady would venture forth during the day without a well-fitting pair of leather gloves. For evening parties and balls, she would wear long, elegant white gloves with little pearl buttons at the wrist, because no lady would dance without her gloves on (all that over-exciting skin contact). There would be a second pair in reserve for when the first got soiled and sweaty.

Then came manicures, polished nails and a more relaxed attitude towards naked hands, and out went the social glove, except for State Openings of Parliament and Coronations (and how many of those are pencilled into your diary?) Gloves are for keeping your hands warm. Well-fitting leather gloves are still the ladylike option; don't wear amusing mittens or ski gloves if you're out to impress.

Well-fitting gloves and boots, things of small moment in themselves, tell of a neat and refined taste.

Routledge's Manual of Etiquette,
late nineteenth century.

Shoes

It's blindingly obvious, I know ... but you've got to be able to walk in your shoes. Ladies do not teeter or totter; they glide, confidently. Don't buy shoes that pinch or compress your toes. If you've got fat feet, buy wide-fitting shoes. If your heels are a nightmare of dry skin, don't wear sling-backs. Ideally, shoes should bend with your foot; totally immobile, rigid soles, such as wedges, make walking any distance difficult.

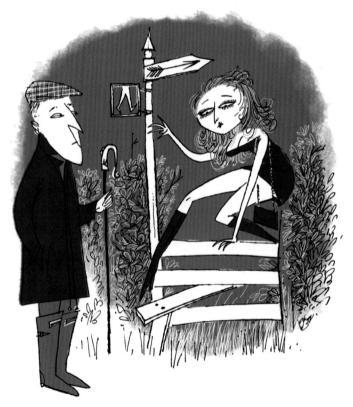

Good shoes can flatter your feet, and good doesn't mean eye-wateringly expensive, it just means well designed, well fitting and well made. Flip-flops are for the beach, as are Crocs, although some might say they would be better off thrown in the bin. Fashion boots with heels are for walking in town, not stumbling along country lanes or over fields. Walking boots, Wellington boots and riding boots should be well made and fit properly.

Ladies are sensible people who know all this. They know that shoes should be fit for purpose, and they know how to look after them, too. So take your common sense shoe-shopping and invest in shoe polish, shoe brushes, shoe trees and all that stuff. You know it makes sense.

Ladies do not teeter or totter;
they glide, confidently ... Good
shoes can flatter your feet, and
good doesn't mean eye-
wateringly expensive.

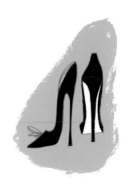

Jewellery

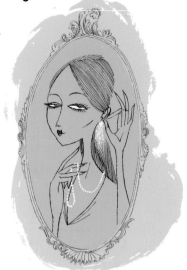

Anything sparkly and precious should be worn only in the evening and kept in the bank during the day. As a general rule, ladies don't do über-bling or vulgar. Big sparkly earrings are teamed with an understated necklace, or even no necklace at all, and a glorious necklace may be offset with small earrings. Precious brooches should always complement the outfit, and size and bling-factor should be taken into consideration when deciding what additional jewels to wear. For those without proper jewels, contemporary pieces have the same sort of impact, so it makes sense to let one lovely piece shine rather than clutter yourself up like an avant-garde junkyard.

Daytime jewels should be discreet: a little silver necklace, a string of pearls, that sort of thing. As far as fake jewellery goes, if you're big, wear big; if you're small, wear small.

As a general rule, ladies don't do über-bling or vulgar.

Hair And Make-Up

Ladies have easy-to-manage hair that is beautifully cut, swishily clean, flattering to the face and discreetly coloured. The rest of us are on an endless search for a hairdresser who can perform miracles. A few unladylike no-nos spring to mind: fake-hair hairbands; over-ornate up-dos; plaits on the middle-aged; fiddling with your hair or scratching your scalp.

Make-up should flatter and emphasise either the eyes or the lips, but not both. Too much make-up is unladylike and ageing. Daytime make-up should tend towards the no-make-up look, which requires both skill and practice. After dark you can segue into brilliant lips or brilliant eyes, but never both. Too much lip gloss suggests 'porn star'. Over-plucked eyebrows look a bit tacky, too – in fact, they'd go very nicely thank you with the overdone up-do. Repair your make-up in private, not in public.

Tattoos And Body Piercing

Don't. Just don't.

> **Here's a tip for hair:** Get brushing. In privileged circles, lady's maids would brush their mistresses' hair at the end of the day – at least a hundred soothing strokes with a proper bristle brush. This is a haircare routine that actually works, stimulating the scalp and distributing natural oils, not just a bit of business gratuitously inserted into period dramas so the characters can exchange gossip and advance the plot.

All The Gear But No Idea

Dressing for sport is a tricky one. You need the right gear, but you don't want to dress in excess of your talent. Some time ago, when rollerblading was the thing, I was much amused to see a whole family of smart Italians emerge from Daddy's sleek limo, all kitted out with brand new top-of-the-range helmets and boots, colour-co-ordinated velvet track suits, cashmere leg warmers, knee pads, elbow pads, ergonomic water bottles … A few tentative steps into the elegant tree-lined avenues of Parco Montagnolo in Bologna and they all fell flat on their noses and couldn't get up. It was great for the spectators, but not a moment for the family album. So bear that little scenario in mind when choosing gym outfits, tennis stuff, ski gear, etc.

Deportment

You can be decked out from head to toe in the most divine ensemble, but if you ain't got the poise and posture, babe, you're nowhere. Head up, shoulders back, tummy in, back straight and

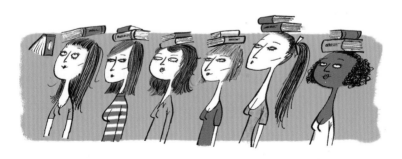

walk from the hips. Practice makes perfect, which explains all those old-fashioned finishing-school images of gels walking around with books balanced on their heads.

Exercises can help. Natural ladylike deportment comes from riding horses, curtseying to royalty and taking ballet lessons, but Pilates is a good alternative for the modern girl because it, too, is all about holding your body upright. Here are just two exercises to kick-start your awareness of your posture.

The roll down Stand up straight, place your feet hip-distance apart, with your chin parallel to the floor and your arms relaxed by your side. Inhale deep into your ribs and hold your tummy in. Exhale and, letting your arms hang heavy, lower your chin towards your chest and keep going, vertebra by vertebra, until your hands touch the floor (if you can). Inhale. Exhale and roll up again, vertebra by vertebra, until you are standing tall. Repeat until you can feel what standing tall means.

The dumb waiter This exercise is to make you aware of holding your shoulders back and down. You can even do this sitting at your desk to ease 'computer hunch'. Hold your upper body upright, and your head high, shoulders back and down, elbows tucked in to your waist, forearms parallel to the ground as if holding a tray, palms up. Inhale. As you exhale, keeping your elbows pinned in to your waist, slowly rotate your forearms outwards as far as they can go, thus pulling your shoulder blades together and down, making your neck long and swanlike. Inhale. Exhale to bring the arms back very, very slowly. You can do this with a rubber exercise band to increase resistance.

Sitting Down

For a proper ladylike look, keep your knees together and your
ankles crossed, and lean slightly to one side. Above all, don't
fidget, don't kick your shoes off or put your feet on the table, and
don't slump in your chair like a half-filled sack of walnuts.

Getting Out of a Car While Wearing a Skirt

A useful skill that does require practice. The movements should
flow and look effortless.

Step one: Prepare by pulling your skirt down as far as you can.
If wearing a long enough skirt, pull it down to cover your knees,
and push excess fabric away from the car door so that it doesn't
impede your exit. You are going to need both hands for this
manoeuvre, so give your handbag and shopping to someone
wearing trousers.

Step two: Open the car door … or smile sweetly as it is opened
for you.

Step three: Put your feet on the ground, keeping your knees
firmly together.

Step four: Swivel hips and upper body to follow legs.

Step five: Push up, either with both hands on the seat or one
hand to the rear of the seat as you use the other hand to keep
your skirt down or accept a helping hand. Start to rise smoothly.

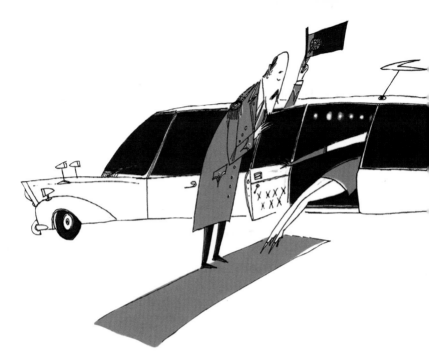

Step six: DUCK! Or rather, dip your head elegantly under the doorframe so you don't knock yourself out.

Step seven: Check the feet. Make sure your feet are on stable ground, which is tricky in high heels, and that you can see where you are going to take your first step. You don't want to do all this elegant stuff and then fall flat on your nose.

Step eight: Bottom out last. Unfold, smile and step away.

To get into a car, reverse the order. Bottom goes in first, head dips, knees swivel round. It is advisable to open the car door before starting this reverse manoeuvre.

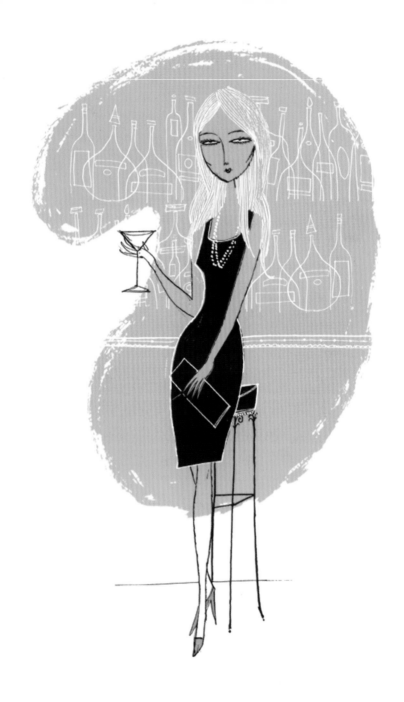

Chapter 2

How to Act Like a Lady

*Be pretty if you can,
be witty if you must,
but be gracious
if it kills you.*

Elsie de Wolfe (1865–1950),
American actress and best-dressed socialite, who
moved in all the right circles and invented interior
design and the cocktail party.

The Communal Spirit

Let us start with table manners, because if you can make yourself agreeable at the dinner table, you are halfway up the social ladder. Back in the misty depths of civilisation, the main social function of the family, tribe or clan was to come together to share a feast of woolly mammoth *à la plancha*. Customs evolved to ensure that everyone was fed according to rank and need, the hunters were accorded suitable respect, and stories or experiences that might affect the well-being of the tribe were exchanged. ('Sharpen your spears, guys – herd of buffalo approaching from the north!')

If you think about it, apart from napkins, knives and forks, tables, chairs and endless books on etiquette, not much has changed, really. A person with good table manners is someone who embraces the communal spirit at every level, from arriving on time so that others don't have to wait, through being pleasant to be with, to making good conversation. ('There's a brilliant new butcher specialising in buffalo steaks opening soon on the North End Road!')

At Table

Manners are not just for best. If you respect your friends and family, you will appear at the table when called (not 20 minutes late) and you won't submit them to off-putting sights of a full mouth chewing, horrible sprawling posture, grabbing food, texting, tweeting and fidgeting. Imagine how the person who made the effort to put the meal on the table is going to feel about that. It's very important to keep the cook happy, since an angry, resentful cook is a dangerous enemy.

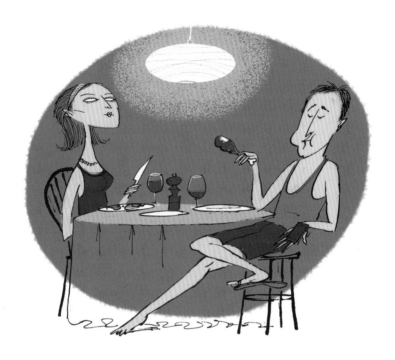

These are the basics: leave all communications devices, apart from your brain, switched off and preferably in another room. Sit up straight, pass food to others before helping yourself, and don't grab. Say please and thank you. Don't reach across; ask for things to be passed. Don't use your own cutlery in a communal dish; use the serving spoon provided. Don't drown your food with seasoning or sauces before tasting it or you risk upsetting the cook (unwise – see opposite).

Leave all communications devices,
apart from your brain, switched off.

Food Intolerances, Yours or Anyone Else's

This is a party, for heaven's sake. If you are a committed vegetarian or you are aware that certain foods actually make you sick, tell your hostess in advance and *don't bring the subject up at table*. If you are not a regular visitor to the household and the cook has forgotten to take your problems into account, muddle through as best you can, leaving the bits you can't eat on the side of your plate.

Take medicines before you arrive and not at the dinner table: it's a real downer watching someone counting out hypertension pills when everyone's in the mood for a party.

Ready, Steady, Go!

Before embarking on your meal, shake out your napkin and put it on your lap. When bread is handed round, you can start eating it straight away, but don't devour it as if you haven't eaten in months. If the food served is cold (a salad starter, for instance), wait for everyone to be served and sitting down before starting. If the food is hot, the host(ess) will often urge you to start, and you should, but not until the host and hostess are at least seated.

{ **A tip:** If your hostess has decorated the table with dry-clean-only napkins made from stiff gauzy purple chiffon and tied about in Martha Stewart fashion with tendrils of ivy and barbed wire, behave as badly as you like to ensure that you don't get invited again. As a rule of thumb, the prissier the napkin and the fussier the table setting, the worse the food. }

Eating Neatly

Don't shovel food into your mouth. Convey it from plate to mouth with a fork, and don't eat peas (or anything else, for that matter) from your knife. Don't gobble and don't pick, and do try to eat quietly. A person talking with a mouthful of food is a dreadful thing to behold.

Napkin Know-how

Put it in your lap, not tucked into your cleavage. Use it to dab greasy lips before drinking wine, to wipe fingers and to dry them after a dabble in the finger bowl, and to catch drips. If you leave the table during the meal, leave your napkin on your seat, not in full view on the table. It goes on the table – not folded, but decently bunched up to hide unsightly stains – at the conclusion of the meal.

A Dinner Party

This is an opportunity to be at your ladylike best. Make an effort to look nice – it's respectful to your hosts. Get into the communal spirit by offering a contribution: bring wine, flowers or food-related goodies, such as chocolate or a lovely olive oil. Be thoughtful with the gift, though; rather nothing than a bottle of cheap and nasty, a Snickers bar or a bunch of wilting carnations from a garage forecourt.

Fashionably Late

If you are invited for a meal, don't arrive early in case you catch the host or hostess in the shower or stashing away the carry-out cartons, making for an awkward social moment. Arrive no later than ten minutes after the stated time. More than 30 minutes late is straying into 'I'll be there when it suits me' territory: very bad manners.

Which Knife?

A lady must exude confidence. Hovering uncertainly over the cutlery, darting nervous glances around the table to see how other people intend to manage, is a dead give-away. If the table is properly laid, you can confidently work from the outside in. If the selection of cutlery or the food placed in front of you is daunting in any way, delay making any crucial cutlery decisions by embarking on some witty tale involving hand gestures until your host(ess) has set an example. You never know, they might have been given a set of Georgian silver asparagus tongs as a wedding present and the whole table will be doomed to grapple and fiddle with the stupid things. A lady will take this in her stride, and make a mental note to be out of town the next time an invitation presents itself in the asparagus season.

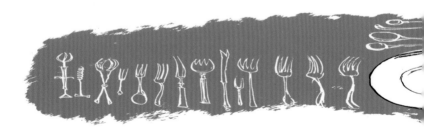

Stones And Bones

Something in your mouth that shouldn't be there? Cup your hand over your mouth, eject the article and discreetly place it on the side of your plate. Nobody noticed, did they?

Holding Your Knife And Fork

Please don't hold your knife like a pen. It's very wrong and, along with grasping a fork like a dagger, a sure signifier that you belong in outer social darkness. That can be quite a fun and funky place, of course, but if you've gone to the bother of buying this book, you clearly want to escape, so pay attention. Tuck the handle into your palm, with your index finger along the top and your thumb on one side of the handle. The same goes for the fork, with prongs facing downwards, although if you're eating using only a fork, then it's prongs upwards.

If soup is served in a flat bowl with a rim, the spoon motion goes away from you to the outer rim so that you convey the full spoon over the soup (in case of drips) before continuing the journey to your mouth. Don't overfill the spoon or slurp as you drink from the side of the spoon. If the soup is in a little, deep bowl, it'll probably be full of interesting bits, so just scoop and eat as tidily as you can. Don't pick up the bowl.

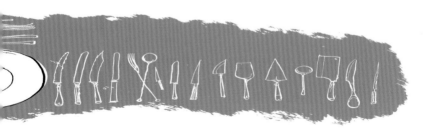

Italians eat spaghetti with a practised twirl of the fork, just loading on enough pasta for one tidy mouthful. There's no shame in using a spoon to steady the fork as you twirl.

Cutlery Semaphore

In the United Kingdom and most of Europe: when you have finished, leave your knife and fork parallel on the 12 o'clock/ 6 o'clock axis, handles towards you, the blade of the knife turned in and the tines of the fork facing up. In America, the knife and fork go on the 10 o'clock/4 o'clock axis with the tines turned down.

In France the convention is completely different: the table is laid with the tines of the fork face down to show off the family crest of entwined initials (𝕴𝕶€𝕬) on the back of the fork. Up, down – does anyone care? Does any of this really matter? Answers on a postcard, please.

Manners are a sensitive awareness of the feelings of others. If you have that awareness, you have good manners, no matter what fork you use.

Emily Post (1872–1960), American writer on etiquette. She started writing after her marriage ended because of her husband's infidelities with a string of chorus girls, which suggests that Miss Manners might have been beautifully behaved but was perhaps not a whole lot of fun.

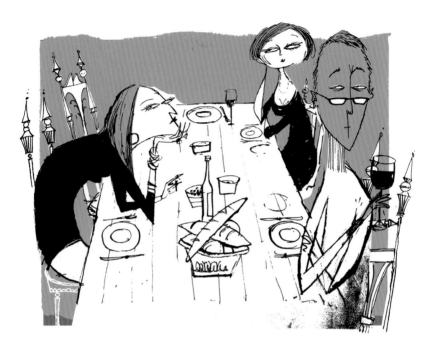

Topics of Conversation

They used to say don't talk about sex, religion or politics, but that prohibition would make for a very dull gathering. What is distasteful (and boring) is banging on about your sex life, your religious beliefs and your personal political ideology. No one wants a sermon or an X-rated guide to what turns you on. Don't preach, do invite contributions, and listen more than you talk, otherwise you will be addressing a collection of extremely bored guests staring glumly into space.

Possibly the dullest thing to talk about at table, aside from house prices and how brilliant or amusing your children are, is diets. When they're eating, people don't want to talk about fasting or the benefits to the upper colon of wheatgrass juice.

Eating With Your Fingers

It is possible to eat a banana with a knife and fork, but quite frankly if you're hanging out with people who are a) that cheapskate about pudding, and b) so uptight that they can't pick up a banana, my advice is to find new friends.

Eating with your fingers is perfectly acceptable when it's done in a ladylike way. The aim is to create as little mess as possible. Wait for the food to cool down; don't blow on it. Don't hunch over your plate, and keep those elbows off the table. Do not eat 'upright' foods as if auditioning for a porn movie. Dispatch hot dogs, asparagus spears and the aforementioned banana with small, decisive bites, put the food down between mouthfuls, and don't wave half-eaten hot dogs in your neighbour's face. Afterwards, don't lick your fingers; use your napkin.

Eating Canapés

This should be done in one mouthful. If the item looks unbalanced or too tricky to manage, let it pass and wait for something less challenging to come round. Don't take more than one from a proffered plate; it signals greed and/or desperation.

Time your canapé eating with your conversation, so that you bite and swallow while listening attentively to your fellow guests explaining how they got here in spite of roadworks blocking the main road into town. Then, when the time comes to reply, you can confidently deliver a sparkling exit line without spraying pastry crumbs, before whirling off stylishly to chase the drinks tray and find more interesting people to talk to.

Tricky Foodstuffs

Asparagus Eat with your fingers, unless the spears are thin and wobbly or drippy with sauce, in which case use a knife and fork.

Cheese If you're cutting your own cheese from the cheese-board, respect the shape of the cheese. If it's round, cut into it like a cake; if it's a wedge, take a 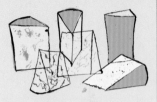 wedge from the wedge. Do not cut off the nose (the point of the wedge), which is the best bit and should be shared.

Crabs Much the same as lobster (see page 42), only much fiddlier. Dressed crabs are a blessing.

Fish on the bone Cut down the centre of the fish, then (attacking one side at a time) run the flat of your knife between the flesh and the bone, easing the fillet on to your plate. Be aware that many fish have little bones all around the outside edge. Tease these out and discard. Now gently lift the whole skeleton – head, tail and backbone – in one elegant movement on to the discard plate. Tuck in only when you've separated the fish from its skeleton and cleared

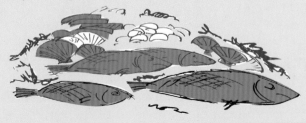

your plate of bones. In a restaurant, the waiter should do all this for you, but you can't expect your host(ess) to fillet individual fish for a tableful of people. Fish cooked on the bone tastes delicious, so it is worth the effort.

Globe artichokes served whole These are delicious, but frankly it's a bit of a penance to get though to the good bits. You may wish to question your host(ess)'s motives for presenting you with such a tricky, prickly dish. Strip off the outer leaves one by one, dip the tiny, fleshy lump at the bottom of the leaf into the melted butter or whatever dip is provided, then delicately strip the edible bit with your teeth. Pile up the leaves neatly in a discard bowl or on the side of your plate as you go. When you get to the centre leaves, you should be able to pull them off in one go, since there's not much flesh on them to enjoy. Now the choke is revealed: a hairy and inedible crown that tops the prized heart. Pull and scrape this off, discard, then enjoy the delicious, hard-won disc.

Lobster With every lobster, you should get a lobster pick (which looks like something a dental hygienist might have left behind) and a pair of claw crackers. The lobster on your plate will be halved, so there's no problem accessing the flesh in the shell and eating it with your knife and fork. The claws are the best bit, and to get at the flesh you have to crack them open, pull down on the 'thumb' to open them up a bit more, then use the pick to tease out every last edible morsel. It's hard to be prissy and uptight while sharing a lobster feast, as it is a gloriously messy business, involving finger bowls, dripping butter and bits of shell firing off here and there.

Mussels Forks are rather clumsy for extracting mussels from their shells. Mussels are best eaten using an empty shell as a pincer to pull out the flesh. Pile shells in the discard bowl and use a finger bowl to clean up when you've finished.

Oysters Use the little fork to detach the oyster from its half-shell, then put the fork down, pick up the oyster and deliver it direct into your mouth via the wide end. You don't have to swallow them whole: a light bite will increase the pleasure of the experience, which is 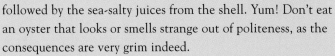 followed by the sea-salty juices from the shell. Yum! Don't eat an oyster that looks or smells strange out of politeness, as the consequences are very grim indeed.

Quail and other small birds Cut off the legs and wings, then slice off the breast bits and eat them with your knife and fork. In relaxed company, you may pick up the legs and nibble at them. Pulling apart the carcass and attacking it with your teeth is medieval, however, and considered unladylike.

Shell-on cooked prawns Off with its head first, then pull apart the legs, releasing the body from the shell. Pull off the tail shell. Prawns and shrimp have to eat, and what looks like a vein running along the back of the beast is the alimentary tract. However unsightly this may look, once cooked it makes little difference to the taste or hygiene of the mouthful. Deveining prawns at the table can be a messy business, so if it doesn't come out easily, forget about it; just eat and enjoy.

Drinking Wine

Wine is the most healthful
and most hygienic of beverages.

Louis Pasteur (1822–1895),
French chemist and microbiologist.

Social rules regarding wine-drinking are designed to *slow you down*. When you are offered a glass, **don't** knock it back in one, wipe your mouth on the back of your hand and wave your empty glass in the direction of the bottle. **Do** hold your glass by the stem, look down into it in a knowledgeable sort of way, swirl the wine gently, sip, savour, say it's delicious and move the conversation briskly along. It's best not to get bogged down in wine-upmanship. If seated at table, put your glass down between sips.

Drinking Too Much Wine

Ladies can behave as disgracefully as they like at parties as long as they know everyone worth knowing and do not have parsley stuck in their teeth.

Choosing Wine

If it is up to you to choose the wine in a restaurant, consult the list to see if there's something there you know you like. If the list is ludicrously long, just ask the waiter. If it's a small restaurant with

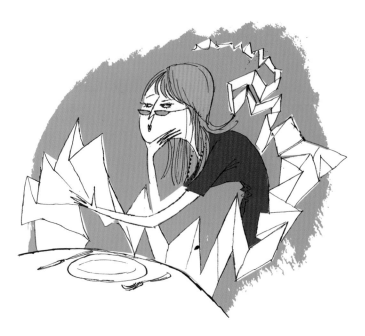

a small wine list, they'll have chosen the wines to go with their food and will know what is the closest to your requirements. In very expensive places, choose the house wine if in doubt – it's not going to be horrid. The waiter will pour a small amount into your glass. Taste it to see if it's the right temperature. Swirling, sniffing and gargling are not called for and will only make the waiter snigger behind your back. These days, thanks to screw tops and plastic corks, wines are rarely 'corked'; if this has happened, the aroma of damp, musty cardboard should alert you instantly.

Pouring Wine

Twist the bottle slightly at the end of the pour to prevent drips, and never fill glasses to the brim. Red wine glasses should be one-third full, white wine glasses half-full and sparkling wine glasses

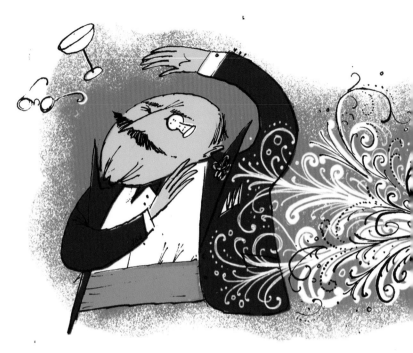

three-quarters full.

Opening Champagne

Everyone, posh or not, needs to know how to do this properly. The champagne should be chilled and the bottle should ideally have rested for a while, as a bottle that has been agitated in transit or shaken vigorously by a 'hilarious' joker pretending to be a racing driver will surely take its revenge.

Step one: Remove the foil. Make sure you have a champagne flute to hand.

Step two: Point the bottle away from people and priceless

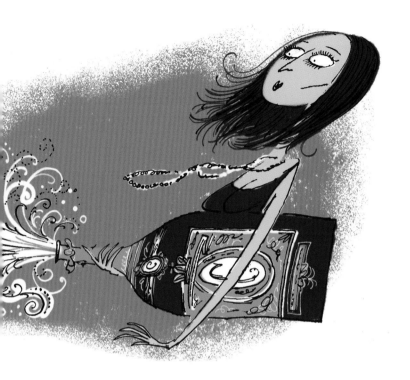

possessions as you loosen the wire cage and discard it, keeping a thumb on the top of the cork.

Step three: Hold the cork firmly with one hand, and twist the bottle (not the cork) very gently with the other. The cork should ease its way out with a sigh, and as the champagne gushes out, your standby flute will come in handy.

Step four: Pour a small amount into each glass and then top up as the bubbles subside. Hold the glass by the stem so the wine isn't affected by the heat of your hands on the body of the glass. Cheers!

Some Useless Information

- You can buy champagne in quarter and half bottles, which are useful for surprise breakfasts or picnics. Winston Churchill had specially made 60-cl (1-pint) bottles of Pol Roger delivered to him at 11 am every day.

- A bottle of champagne, like all bottles of wine, contains 75 cl (1¼ pints).

- A magnum is the equivalent of two bottles.

- A jeroboam is the equivalent of four bottles.

- A rehoboam contains six bottles.

- A methuselah contains eight bottles.

- A salmanazar contains 12 bottles.

- A balthazar contains 16 bottles.

- A nebuchadnezzar contains 20 bottles.

Giant bottles have novelty value, but because they are too big to manage during the second fermentation, most champagne houses carry out the fermentation in magnums and then decant into the larger bottles. For that reason, you don't get the full fizz pressure and there's more chance of oxidation. The ladylike conclusion is that bubbly in ridiculouly large bottles is best left to show-offs who have been doing weight training: a full nebuchadnezzar weighs in at more than 38 kilos (about 83 lb).

Drinking Spirits

A lady should know just what she wants when it comes to ordering spirits and cocktails, rather than simpering in a girly way: 'Oh, just something fruity with a straw for little me!' Know which cocktails you like, but if you wish to impress, don't go for anything with a parasol and/or a sparkler or a name stiff with *double entendre*.

The purpose of a pre-dinner **aperitif** is to stimulate the appetite and the conversation. Champagne or dry white wine are good; if you're offered spirits, choose clear over dark, and if in doubt, stick to a martini or a gin-and-tonic. G&Ts are getting quite exciting, with interesting gins and flavoured alcoholic liqueurs, such as elderflower or cassis. This may even be the Year of the Gin-and-Tonic – it's definitely revival time. A **digestif** is an after-dinner drink designed to put you to sleep, and is generally a dark spirit, such as a brandy, Armagnac or whisky, served neat.

Some Helpful Cocktail Terms:

Highball is a drink served over ice in a tall glass, made from a spirit with a larger amount of non-alcoholic mixer. So a gin-and-tonic is technically a highball, as is a whisky-and-ginger.

Straight up refers to a mixed drink that has the ice strained out of it as it is poured into the glass.

Neat means an unmixed spirit served without ice.

Martini was originally very, very chilly gin with a whisper of dry vermouth and an olive. Now the vodka martini is just as common, so it is best to specify your spirit.

Making The Perfect Gin-and-tonic

A lady should be able to do one thing superbly well in every field of endeavour. Here's how to make the perfect G&T.

You will need the following:

- Decent gin – one with character, such as Bombay Sapphire, Sipsmiths or Hendricks.
- A small bottle of the finest organic tonic water you can lay your hands on (Fever-Tree is a good make). Big bottles go flat between pours, and are therefore best avoided. Good tonic is vital for this enterprise; it should be refreshing and slightly bitter, and taste of quinine. You may also require a bottle-opener.
- A large highball glass.
- A lime, a sharp knife and a cutting board.
- Ice, made from distilled water, straight from the freezer.
- A long-handled spoon.

First, deal with the lime. Roll it forwards and backwards under your hand on the board to break down the membranes within and get the juice flowing. Now cut it in half through the circumference, and cut each half into four wedges.

Gently squeeze a wedge of lime into the glass; throw in the wedge. Pour in a double measure of gin (about 50 ml or 2 fl oz).

Fill the glass with ice and muddle it with the spoon.

Open the tonic and pour about 150 ml (5 fl oz) into the glass, then give it a couple of stirs with the spoon.

Add more ice if the glass doesn't look generously full, and float a second lime wedge on top.

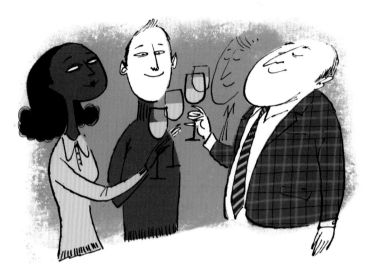

Toasting And Clinking

So here we are: lots of people gathered together, usually for a reason, and it seems right to acknowledge the occasion and say 'cheers'. All very convivial. The person making the toast – normally the host(ess) – will raise a glass to the health, wealth and happiness of the assembled company. That is the cue for all to repeat the toast before clinking glasses with neighbours and taking a celebratory sip. Don't clink if the host doesn't clink, and don't clink in a crowd of 500; you'll be at it all day.

Why Clink?

Back in medieval times, when wine was cloudy and life was cheap, a vigorous clinking of goblets was a sign of trust between friends that no one's mug of wine had been poisoned. In a gathering of distrustful acquaintances, it created the chance for wine to spill from one chalice to another and spread the risk. Today it's about trust and friendship. If you clink, you should look into the eyes of your co-clinker.

Toasting Tips

A host will sometimes toast the assembled company at the beginning of the meal. After the main course has been cleared, it's open season, and, if the mood is right, a guest may feel moved to raise a toast to the host or to some collective enterprise. All should then raise their glasses, murmur the toast and sip. Once you've clinked, you've clinked, and there's no need to keep bashing the glassware.

If the toast is specifically directed to one person – 'To Arabella, for climbing Mount Everest!', for example – Arabella remains seated and smiles sweetly as the assembled company stands up (or maybe doesn't), raises glasses and mumbles 'To Arabella' before sipping. Arabella does not sip; she must not drink to herself.

Formal Toasting

Very formal dinners, in banqueting halls with everyone in full evening dress, have their own microclimate of behaviour that has nothing to do with the real world. Toasts and speeches are more the point of the affair than the food and drink, so just go with the flow: smile, bow, stand, clap, sit and raise your glass when others do. And for goodness' sake, do try to keep awake. Be aware that toast usually follows toast, so don't drain your glass at the very beginning or you'll have nothing to look forward to as time drags painfully by.

Dancing

Don't take to the dance floor with a cigarette or a drink. Try not to flail about, and don't bombard the DJ with requests. The golden rule is that the dance floor is not all about you.

If you've been invited to a formal ballroom-y affair (a charity ball or a work-related shindig), I advise taking a few lessons in fox-trotting and samba and suchlike, and learning to dance as part of a couple. NB: Tall young ladies who went to girls' schools where such social skills as ballroom dancing were on the curriculum may find that all those years 'being the man' have left them at a disadvantage in the real world. It's time to find a taller partner, stop steering and learn to do it going backwards.

The thing to do is fit in. If everyone is gliding about in waltz time, don't attempt a wild break-dance improvisation as it will put the other dancers off their stride (see the golden rule, above).

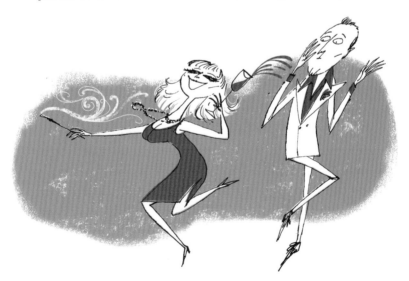

How to Act Like a Lady **53**

The thing to do is fit in. If everyone is gliding about in waltz time, don't attempt a wild break-dance improvisation.

If the dance floor is crowded, weave your way around as seamlessly as possible without resorting to battering-ram tactics. Fancy steps, over-complex moves, aerial lifts and dropping surprisingly to the floor are okay for professional dancers performing an exhibition, but could be construed as taking the piss at the Dental Hygienists' Association Annual Dinner and Dance.

Dancing at Weddings

Traditionally the newly married couple, as guests of honour, dance the first dance together, and everyone stands around choked up with the romance of it all, then gradually joins in. For the second dance, the bride dances with her father and the groom with his mother (presuming the old folk have been invited).

Scottish Dancing

These set dances are splendid fun, and knowing how to do them is one of those skills a proper lady just has. It comes with the territory, thanks to thundering round the gym to the strains of the Gay Gordons at girls' private schools. If you missed out on this, you can teach yourself with a DVD, but it's better to take lessons. Strip the Willow and the Dashing White Sergeant are both a good laugh, featuring full-on galloping, whirling and stamping. What's not to like? Scottish country dancing is also a good aerobic workout.

Vomiting

If you start to feel woozy or unwell, grab a napkin, *leave the room at once* and head for the WC or out into the street, holding the napkin over your mouth. Obviously, it's best to vomit into a lavatory bowl, but if it's got to be behind a bush, then so be it. If there is no way you can clean yourself up, it's best to slip off to the nearest taxi rank. If you feel better and suddenly able to cope, then freshen up, gargle with water and repair your make-up. Explain your absence by saying that you had to make an emergency phone call. Never complain, and never explain the real reason.

What everyone agreed was not very nice, was the way Clémence had carried on. Obviously, she wasn't the kind of girl you'd ask again: she'd ended up showing off everything she'd got, and she'd puked all down one of the muslin curtains and completely ruined it. At least the men went into the street to do it; Lorilleux and Poisson, when they felt queer, managed to dash as far as the pork-butcher's shop. Breeding always tells.

Émile Zola, *L'Assommoir* (1877)

> **A little tip:** If you need to sober up, it's time to stop drinking. Try holding your wrists (palms up) under cold running water. I don't know if this has any physiological effect, but it does regroup the mind, and gives you a chance to say severely to yourself: I'm far too drunk, it's time to go home.

Travelling Like a Lady

When travelling with someone,
take large doses of patience and tolerance
with your morning coffee.

Helen Hayes (1900–1993), multi award-winning
actress who knew a thing or two about travelling.

Taxis

A lady should always carry taxi money hidden about her person so she can make a swift exit from any sticky situation. Hail a cab by waving while leaning out from the pavement to get the driver's attention. Whistling and yelling won't help as a) the cab driver probably won't hear you from inside his cab with the radio on and b) he/she will probably ignore you as a risky ride and pick someone better behaved. Tell the driver where you want to go before you get in the cab and be prepared for the possibility of having to give directions. Tipping is a debatable issue. In the US it is usually expected and can be anywhere from 15–25 percent. In the UK and Europe, it's up to you to add what you wish— 10 percent of the fare would please most drivers.

Public Transport

Please, no loud conversations on mobile phones. Nothing is more enraging to fellow passengers than being forced to listen to a one-sided conversation. Ladies do not enrage. And why is it that you always find yourself sitting next to the non-stop motormouth?

Presumably someone somewhere else is listening to the uninterested person on the other end of this conversation whisper the occasional 'Yah!', 'Must have been awful' and 'Oh, poor you!', which, while irritating, is not quite as bad as the full, shouty, blow-by-blow drama.

A lady notices the needs of fellow passengers, and moves her bag from the seat next to her if she sees someone hoping to sit down. She smiles, keeps her legs and arms to herself, and passes the journey either looking dreamily out of the window recalling those precious stolen moments with the gamekeeper in the woods, or reading an improving novel.

A lady knows that eating smelly, messy, greasy food in the confines of a train or bus is just not done. If the journey is long, it is to be hoped that she will have had the foresight to ask the butler to pack her a pretty and uncontroversial picnic – some

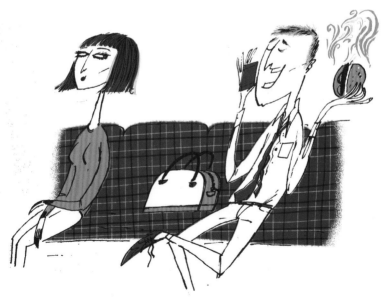

cucumber sandwiches, perhaps, and a flask of cold soup, with maybe a bunch of grapes, a square or two of good-quality chocolate and a great big linen napkin to catch all the crumbs.

Air Travel

This is mostly unspeakable, unless you're travelling first class. In the back of the bus all passengers are equal and entitled to recline their seats (thoughtfully) and to claim space on at least one armrest. The worst thing is to be sitting next to 'a people person' who wants to tell you his or her life story. Don't be that person, and if you find yourself sitting next to the plane bore, use every trick in the body-language repertoire: don't make eye contact, bury your nose in a book and plug in your headphones. The next worst thing is sitting in the midst of a rowdy group. You can always ask to be moved: the staff may ignore you, and they probably will, but no one will kill you for asking.

Driving

Real born ladies should be accomplished at driving four-wheel-drive cars full of dogs over muddy fields on Daddy's estate. They also need to know how to park outside Harvey Nichols, Barney's or Saks and throw the keys to the doorman while exiting a low-slung car with style (see page 28). The rest of us should avoid road-rage situations, perfect our parallel parking, remember not to eat or drink while actually driving, and stop using the rearview mirror for applying make-up while paused at pedestrian crossings.

Many a lady driver is subject to back-seat (or passenger-seat) drivers who give out a stream of instructions, wince, and do that fake-braking thing while covering their eyes and calling loudly upon assorted deities. This kind of behaviour is not only extremely annoying, but also dangerously bad for a lady's concentration. If the back-seat driver cannot be cured of this terrible habit by kind words and reasoned argument, then I suggest putting them in the front seat and forever after refusing to drive them anywhere, especially back from a good night out. That should do the trick.

At The Theatre or Opera

It is not necessary to dress up for the theatre, but it's a good idea to look clean and smart, especially if you're going to eat out afterwards. If you have a bulky overcoat, a rucksack or your weekly shopping, leave it in the cloakroom. Remember that you will be sitting in an auditorium with hundreds of other people who all want to concentrate on the spectacle on the stage, so don't douse yourself in heady perfume, pile your hair up on top of your head and stick a feather in it, or wear jangling jewellery. Arrive in time to order interval drinks and be seated, turn off your phone and don't eat anything. You are there for just a couple of

Applause tips: Clap the conductor as he (or sometimes, but not often enough, she) arrives on the podium, and clap after the overture. If everyone else is clapping after a particularly lovely aria (that's the bit with the tune), join in. Clap like mad at the end. If the performance has been exceptionally dire, it's best not to boo unless you are a real opera buff and you've paid for the tickets.

hours, and every lady knows that it is perfectly possible to sit through an act at least without chomping, chewing or rustling chocolate wrappers to the enormous annoyance of your neighbours. At the interval you can leave your coat or jacket on your chair, and take just your handbag to the crowded bar.

Opera goers are generally divided into two camps: fanatics and the rest of us. If you're there with a fanatic, be prepared: read up on the story so you know what is happening and don't have to ask why X is murdering/hiding from/declaring undying love to Y. Opera stories never make much sense anyway.

Gossip

You could subscribe to the view that if you can't think of anything nice to say, then say nothing. But how dull is that? A gossip session is good for the soul and creates bonds within a group. However, a lady will take care not to say things that are unspeakably vile about someone close, because gossip has a nasty habit of biting back.

Good gossip is dangerous and bold, hinting at secrets you were sworn to carry to the grave. It doesn't matter if you make it all up; it's much more interesting if you can be creative.

Little White Lies

These are the oil that lubricates the wheels of life. No one could live for very long with Little Miss Truthful. A bit of embroidery never did a story any harm, and finding something nice to say in order to avoid hurt feelings is a positively good thing. What do

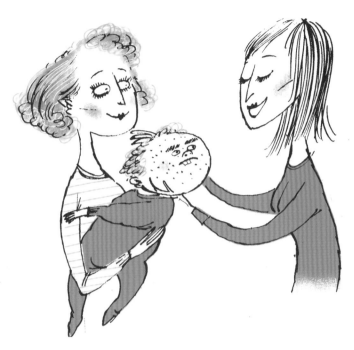

you say to the parents proudly presenting the ugliest baby in the world? Nice hair, lovely eyes, pretty hands … dig deep and you'll find something. Just don't mention the rash.

Excuses are often a good way to ease the path. It's better to say, 'Oh, I'd love to come but I have a doctor's appointment,' than, 'I'm not coming over to your place because the last time I was there your dreadful husband put his hand up my skirt.' Don't elaborate on your excuses – keep them simple. If pressed for why you have a doctor's appointment that can't be missed, just say you'd rather not talk about it; otherwise you'll have to keep track of an imagined disease all the way from diagnosis through treatment to cure.

Basing your life on a lie, on the other hand, is a doomed strategy. Awarding yourself a degree you don't have, or claiming a branch of a family tree that isn't yours, will unravel in the long run. Even lying about your age is fraught with danger; you can't keep relatives and old school friends in the closet forever, and what's going to happen when they start sending you 40th birthday cards when your social group has you down as a mature 29?

> *If you haven't got anything nice to say about anybody, come sit next to me.*
>
> **Alice Roosevelt Longworth** (1884–1980),
> eldest daughter of Theodore Roosevelt
> (26th President of the United States),
> and a committed wild child all her long life.

Social Media

Social media sites, including Twitter, Facebook and Instagram, have created a very useful tool for keeping up with friends and relatives, for marketing and running a business, sourcing the wisdom of crowds and holding tyrants to account. Remember, though, that no one wants to know every intimate and mundane detail of your life. Who, other than a stalker, could possibly be interested in your opinion on colonic irrigation? And remember that any time in thrall to an electronic device is consequently deducted from experiencing life face to face.

A lady should keep her counsel and surround herself with mystery, and so I prefer to keep clear of social networking in general. The only advice I will offer is to do no harm when online.

Introductions

These are dead simple, really, unless you suffer from name amnesia. Speak clearly and look people in the eye. Always introduce the lesser mortal to the higher mortal. The ranks of mortals are as follows: people with titles, old people, women, men. In making the introductions, say the name of the higher mortal first, and then give your introducees a clue about how they should address one another, ensuring that somewhere along the line they get a first name and a last, and, if it's that sort of party, the rank. Last names are not always necessary for friends on first-name and equal terms.

Thus, when introducing your aged Aunt Mildred and your latest lover, do it like this:

"Aunt Mildred, I'd like to introduce you to my friend Sebastian Flyte. Sebastian, this is my aunt, Mrs Piper."

If Sebastian, having made himself charming to Aunt Mildred, now wants to meet your foxy friend Desirée, 'Desirée, this is Sebastian, he's just leaving,' will do fine.

A lady should keep her counsel and surround herself with mystery.

It is helpful to acknowledge relationships between people and to give little hints as to how you are connected. If introducing a single person to a group of people, for instance, you would say: 'Arabella, this is Torquil and Tony, old friends from university, and Tony's partner, Bertrand. Everybody, this is my friend Arabella, who has just climbed Mount Everest.' Then they've all got something to work with.

And who is that approaching? It's a middle-aged archbishop with his eye on converting your Aunt Mildred. 'Your Grace, may I introduce my aunt, Mrs Piper. Aunt Mildred, this is the Archbishop of Gotham City.'

The party is warming up nicely, and what a guest list! Next to the buffet, two elderly men circulate each other warily while

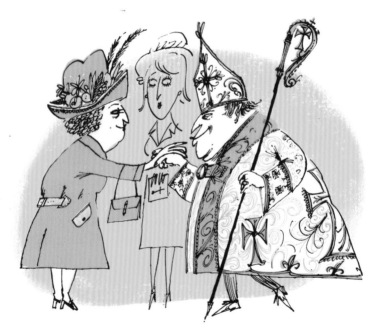

filling their plates. They don't know each other, but you know them both and are unsure which one is the elder. How can it matter? Just pick the one you like best to be the higher mortal, and then drag them over to rescue Aunt Mildred.

Invitations And RSVPs

It's a simple enough rule that the invitation should reflect the event. A stiff piece of white card with gilt edging and engraved script will denote a very formal do, while a group email sends out an altogether different vibe. Every invitation – formal, informal or in-between – should communicate to the guest what to expect and give a clue as to what to wear. That doesn't mean setting out a list; there's a lot you can convey creatively about an event using graphics and tone of voice. Send out invitations to weddings eight to ten weeks in advance, those for catered events where numbers really matter should be sent six weeks ahead, those for birthday parties three weeks in advance, and those for dinner parties or drinks a week or so ahead.

When you receive an invitation, *reply* and stick to your commitment. Fuzzy, bet-hedging 'maybe's are every host(ess)'s nightmare. The reply should be in keeping with the spirit of the invitation, so if you have received a formal invitation to, let's say, a grand and glittering wedding, you should reply accordingly. It's traditional to reply to formal invitations in the third person according to a set format. Why? Because standard wording makes it much easier at the other end to separate the yeses from the nos, and gives reassurance that all the guests know where they are going and when. Setting out on a creative tangent is just annoying. Replies should be prompt, handwritten in fountain pen on proper paper or card, and centred on the page with the date written at the bottom. They should go something like this:

> *Miss Elizabeth Bennet thanks Mr Charles Bingley for his kind invitation to the marriage of his sister Caroline to Fitzwilliam Darcy at St Paul's on Saturday 24th August at 11 o'clock and afterwards at Netherfield Park, but much regrets she is unable to attend/and is delighted to accept.*

Reply to informal invitations in the spirit in which they were extended, bearing in mind the ease of sorting replies at the other end. 'Thanks, we'd love to come!'

Silent gratitude isn't much use to anyone.

Gladys Bronwyn Stern (1890–1973),
prolific English novelist, now mostly out of print.

Thank You

A prompt little note to say thank you for a pleasant stay or a present received is always appreciated. Handwritten is best and a well-chosen card is thoughtful. There's no need to go overboard with gushing letters of thanks if you've just popped over for a drink. A text or an email is just fine to say thanks for dinner.

The Perfect House Guest

She will arrive with a simple, appropriate house gift, ensure that she fits in with the household routine, and know instinctively when to take time out and give the hosts some space. She will also sense when the moment has come to leave. As a guest, it is your duty to turn your radar on so that you can sense these things, and to get the hang of who likes to sit where so you don't plonk yourself in the host's favourite chair and cause resentment. You need to sense the protocol with the newspaper in the morning and the routine for washing dishes. When is breakfast? Do your sleeping/waking habits dovetail with those of your hosts? Is helping yourself to tea/coffee/juice useful or a burden? Always offer assistance at mealtimes, and keep the bathroom clean and your room tidy. If your stay runs into days rather than hours, offer to buy and cook at least one meal or take the hosts out to eat. On leaving, offer to strip the bed and stack all the sheets and used towels in a pile for easy laundering. Get all that down and then concentrate on being a warm, witty, companionable and thoughtful friend, and you'll certainly be asked back.

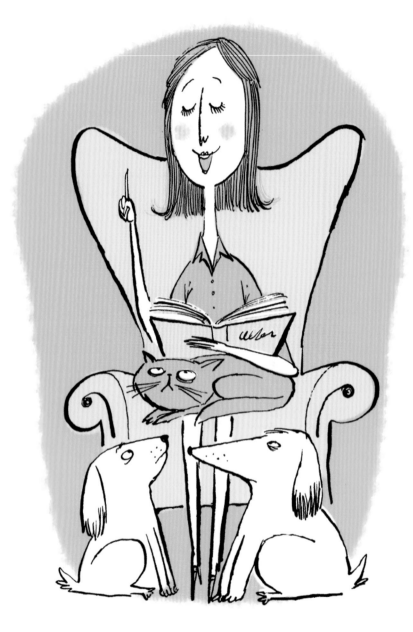

Chapter 3

How to Sound
Like a Lady

———◆———

Speak clearly,
if you speak at all;
Carve every word
before you let it fall.

Oliver Wendell Holmes, Sr. (1809–1894),
American physician, poet and author.

Speaking Properly

You cannot pass for a lady unless you speak properly. But the good news is that anyone with the will to do so can learn to round out their vowels and crisp up their consonants. As many assorted rascals throughout history have discovered, a posh voice is a passport to another world. I'm not suggesting for one moment, dear reader, that your motivation for all this self-improvement is to penetrate High Society and pinch the jewels (but when you are laundering your ill-gotten gains, just remember who got you through the door ...)

Mumbled, unclear, whaddyasay? Back to the scullery with you! You will never catch your prince, Cinderella, or the jewels, unless you sound like convincing princess material. And if the prince proves a disappointment, your new-found cut-glass accent will see you sail through the divorce courts, shine in the media spotlight and open doors to a megabucks job. What is there to lose?

Relax And Breathe ...

A proper voice starts with controlled breath passing through the voice box and vibrating the two bands of tissue that form your vocal cords. Stage actors, public speakers and classical singers are trained to project their voices, but that doesn't mean shouting at people from a stage. It starts with relaxing and breathing, with the aim of effortlessly focusing your voice to a point on the other side of the room. Practise these breathing exercises when you are quite alone, well away from anyone who might pop their head round the door and laugh at you.

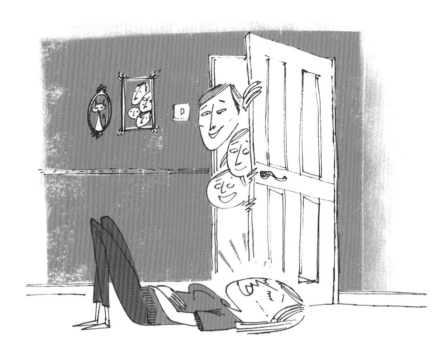

Lie on the floor with your knees bent and your feet flat on the floor. Place your hands on either side of your ribs and fill your lungs so they expand sideways and your hands move out. Breathe in again and exhale for a count of ten. Get a nice rhythm going so your diaphragm gets a bit of a work-out and your brain gets a hit of oxygen. Once you are comfortable with that, vocalise on the out breath with a sustained 'ssshhh', building up to a count of 12. Then hum 'mmmm', which is nice and buzzy on the lips. Then, using your face muscles, start with a hum that opens out into a 12-count vowel sound: 'mmmahhh, mmmooo, mmmeee'. Get used to the feeling of moving your face.

The Muscles of Speech

Your tongue, teeth, lips, roof of the mouth and soft palate are, without getting too technical about it, your organs of speech, and so they need to be in good shape. If you talk with a frozen face and clenched teeth you'll sound the way you look – like a constipated camel.

Start by getting your mouth moving, as if chewing, then yawn with your mouth wide open, then scrunch up your face, hard. Yawn/scrunch, yawn/scrunch … keep going for a bit: it's good for the jawline muscles, too, and you'll thank me later on when all around you, the ugly sisters' jowls start to sag.

Next we move to the lips and tongue. Make a 'brrr' ('I'm freezing') sound with your lips on vibrate. Then say 'la la la la', letting your tongue flick in and out like a lizard. Next, grin and say 'ya ya ya', letting your tongue move against your teeth. Now that your lips and tongue are nicely mobile, it's time for some tongue-twisters. Start slowly, repeating each one as fast and as many times as you can without slurring. If you slur, stop and start again. Ready? Go!

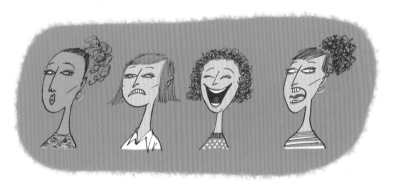

Black bug's blood

A cheap chick sleeps in cheap sheets

Clean clams crammed in clean cans

A dozen double damask dinner napkins

Girl gargoyle, guy gargoyle

Lesser leather never weathered wetter weather better

Red lorry, yellow lorry

Many an anemone sees an enemy anemone

Nine nice night nurses nursing nicely

Rolling red wagons

The sixth sick sheik's sixth sheep is sick

Seventy-seven benevolent elephants

*I'm not the pheasant plucker, I'm the pheasant plucker's
mate. I'm only plucking pheasants 'cause the pheasant
plucker's late.*

*Can you imagine an imaginary menagerie manager
imagining managing an imaginary menagerie?*

And a moving little poem to finish with:

A tree toad loved a she-toad

Who lived up in a tree.

He was a two-toed tree toad

But a three-toed toad was she.

The two-toed tree toad tried to win
The three-toed she-toad's heart,
For the two-toed tree toad loved the ground
That the three-toed tree toad trod.

But the two-toed tree toad tried in vain,
He couldn't please her whim.
From her tree toad bower
With her three-toed power
The she-toad vetoed him.

Essential Pronunciation Guide

Oh, hello! = *airhairlair*

Ask the butler to serve the porridge = *Aarsk the buttler too sarve the porrij*

Your house is very nice = *Yaw hiyce is vair, vair niyce*

I prefer my grouse well hung = *Ei preffer mai growse well hung*

That reminds me: Our gamekeeper is very fit = *Ower gaymekeepah iz vair, vair fitt*

Our family portraits are by Happy Snaps = *Ower femilly pawtrayts are bye Joshoowar Raynulds. Aunt everybody's?*

It's easy to take the piss out of posh, and nobody these days, however posh they are, wants to sound as if they've got a hot potato in their mouth. It's so passé, dahling, to sound the way the Queen did 20 years ago; even the Queen doesn't sound like that any more. Just give words their beginnings, middles and ends, and have regard for the people listening to you. Craft each word before it falls from your lips. English is an absolutely top language with endless vocabulary and lovely rhythms and cadences. Learn to love it. Innit.

Haitch …

… gets an entry all to itself. Dropping aitches and sticking them in the wrong place is, quite simply, not good form. Consider this sentence: *In 'ertford, 'ereford and 'ampshire 'urricanes 'ardly hever 'appen.*

And take this one at speed:
How was Harry hastened so hurriedly from the Hunt?

Most importantly, when reciting the alphabet, the eighth letter is 'aitch' not 'haitch'.

Do not place a light estimate on the art of good reading and good expression.

B.G. Jefferis and **J.L. Nichols**, *Light on Dark Corners: A Complete Sexual Science and a Guide to Purity and Physical Manhood; Advice to Maiden, Wife and Mother; Love, Courtship and Marriage* (1895)

Minding Your Grammar

The lady will, in most cases, have been brought up surrounded by people who can string coherent sentences together, thus absorbing by osmosis sufficient grammar to make even the most banal of utterances speak naturally of good breeding. She will instinctively know her past from her present and future, her subject from her object, her singular from her plural. Speaking grammatically is something a lady needs to be able to do.

There are many delightfully amusing books about grammar that are worthy of further study, but here's a tip for the aspiring lady in a hurry: read aloud, enunciating perfectly. Read good writing, and take your time, relishing the sentence structure, the punctuation, the way thoughts follow thoughts and build to a conclusion.

Warm up with columnists writing for a decent newspaper, journal or such magazines as the *New Yorker* or *Vanity Fair*, or *Practical Fishkeeping* if that's all you can find. In the privacy of your own space, teach yourself to take a breath in preparation, and let the words float out on a controlled column of air (see page 70). Observe how punctuation makes sense of things, how good prose has rhythm, and how comforting it is to know where sentences are going. Good writers and speakers do not waste your time, or theirs, faffing about with 'like … um … to be honest … she was like … you know … and I was like … sort of … yah'.

When stringing together sentences of your own, remember the feel of a well-constructed sentence in your mouth, and take that nanosecond to engage the brain before take-off.

Books delightful to read aloud include anything by Jane Austen, Anthony Trollope and Henry James – and as their plots often hinge on the differences between ladylike and unladylike behaviour, they double as good research. To get the hang of wit and wisdom with panache, the essays of Dorothy Parker, James Thurber and S.J. Perelman are a good starting point. And for a writer who cleverly combines the formality of writing with the informality of speech, search out Caitlin Moran.

Some Things That Really Bug Me

On the subject of the **subject of a sentence**, if you are telling someone about something you did or observed with someone else, you are both the subject of the sentence and you should put the other person first. Not doing so is a dead give-away.

> Example: My *husband and I are enchanted by the exuberant nature of your welcome.*

Take it from the Queen of England. It's not 'Me and Philip are enchanted', is it?

And – leaving Philip out of it – it's not 'Me am enchanted', either. So that's sorted.

Next: **apostrophes**. It's not the remit of this book to bang on about the apostrophe, but for those who wish to abolish it to make the English language 'easier', here's a thought:

> You send a message: 'You're pants.' The response is probably along the lines of: 'You're pretty rubbish yourself and anyway I've slept with your best friend. Goodbye.'

Or perhaps you meant: 'Your pants'? To which you might expect the response: 'Oh really! I so don't remember taking them off and leaving them under your bed! On my way round to pick 'em up, babe!'

Finally: **commas**. 'I've eaten**,** Grandpa' is a kindly way of avoiding an elderly relative's offer of rice pudding. 'I've eaten Grandpa' is a confession that will have you banged up for life.

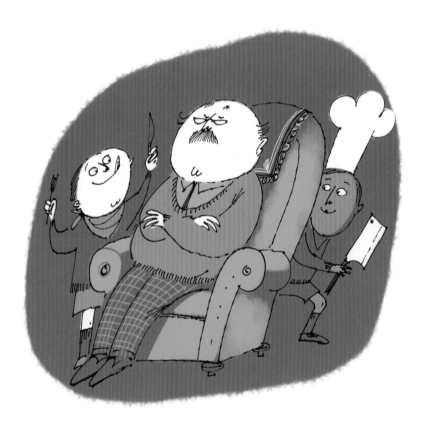

SPOT THE DELIBERATE MISTAKES

Here are some examples of how not to do things:

* Verbs **has** to agree with their subjects.

* Don't use **no** double negatives.

* Never use a preposition to end a sentence **with**.

* **And** don't start a sentence with a conjunction.

* It is wrong to ever split an infinitive except if your mission is **to boldly go** with Mr Spock.

* Avoid clichés **like the plague**.

* Never use a big word when substituting a **diminutive** one would suffice.

Cheerfulness, unaffected cheerfulness, a sincere desire to please and be pleased, unchecked by any efforts to shine, are the qualities you must bring with you into society, if you wish to succeed in conversation.

Arthur Martine,
Martine's Hand-book of Etiquette, and Guide to True Politeness (1866)

Small Talk

Being interesting and interested is the key to success. Let's get the small talk out of the way.

Small-talk tip number one:
Engage the other person with a question or an observation about them. The Queen, who is always well briefed, breaks the ice at garden parties by engaging her awestruck guests thus:

'Have you come far?'

'Overland from Kathmandu, Ma'am.'

'Of course, Arabella, you've just climbed Everest. Jolly good show!'

And then she moves seamlessly on.

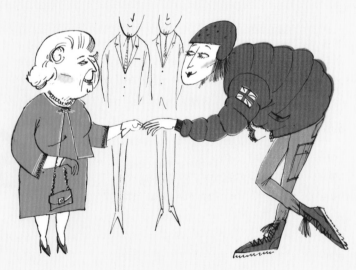

Small-talk tip number two:
Pay attention to the body language of the person, or people, to whom you are speaking. If they are shuffling uncomfortably and gazing into the far distance, you can tell that your line about amateur climbers leaving their dead, frozen friends on the mountain for others to clear up is not going down well, and it's time to change tack.

Small-talk tip number three:
Don't rush to conclusions. Just because Arabella looks uncomfortable at the mention of frozen dead people on mountains doesn't mean she deliberately left them there to die.

Small-talk tip number four:
Don't assume people will agree with you. You may think climbing mountains is a waste of time and effort, but it is highly likely that a professional mountaineer will have a different perspective.

Small-talk tip number five:
Try to learn from every encounter. Arabella has seen things you will never see, and done things you will never do. So shut up and listen to her experiences.

Small-talk tip for Arabella: *Don't over-share.*

Small-talk tip number six:
Do keep up. If you do, you can always talk about the latest trends, topics and breaking news that Arabella may have missed while in the Himalayas. This could open up the conversation to others around you, which could be a blessing after her over-graphic description of frostbitten toes.

The Art of Conversation

With so much electronic interaction available to us within seconds, it's hard to remember what conversations are really for. There's no need to catch up because its highly likely your friends have tweeted, texted, blogged, Instagrammed, Tumblred and Facebooked not only their every move, but also the background and foreground emotional journey of their every move. There's no need to ask what they 'like' because it's up there on various social media websites for all to see. And there's no longer any need to have a merry heated debate about facts – such as which actors lined up for *The Usual Suspects* – because you can look it up on Wikipedia in a trice.

It is perhaps easier to define what conversations should not be rather than what they should be. A series of monologues cannot be classified as a conversation, it's the sound of egos clashing. Likewise, if someone launches into an interminable story, inviting no interaction and determined to get to the end no matter what, that is definitely not a conversation – it's an excellent excuse to go to the lavatory.

Talking and listening, letting minds wander collectively into uncharted waters and down a few ridiculous dead ends is a great way to spend an evening. Much too often, though, even conversations that start out well may get bogged down in the particular: for instance, no one really cares what exactly Arabella did with her Snickers wrappers on the north face of Everest, but the effect of tourism on wild places can open up into lively, more general discussion. A good conversation is bold, inclusive, controversial, interesting and – it is to be hoped – funny.

It's best not to moralise – that's a real downer. Don't dwell on divorce, death or frostbite, either, unless you know the emotional and physical status of everyone in the group. And don't fill every silence with idle chatter.

Real communication is for reaffirming friendships and love, stimulating curiosity, and finding out things about other people. Rules aren't really necessary, but here are a few tips from Cicero (106–43BC) – a portfolio career Roman (philosopher/lawyer/poet/politician/whatever): 'Speak clearly; speak easily but not too much, especially when others want their turn; do not interrupt; be courteous; deal seriously with serious matters and gracefully with lighter ones; never criticise people behind their backs; stick to subjects of general interest; do not talk about yourself; and, above all, never lose your temper.'

In conversation there must be, as in love and in war, some hazarding, some rattling on … so long as you take cheerfulness and good humor for your guides … careful and measured conversation is always, though perfectly correct, extremely dull and tedious – a vast blunder from first to last.

Arthur Martine,
Martine's Hand-book of Etiquette, and Guide to True Politeness (1866)

Foreign Phrases

If using foreign phrases in an English sentence, the lady will use the anglicised pronunciation. Absurd attempts at throaty, spitty Spanish when talking of guerrilla gardening, for instance, are beyond pretentious, as is referring to Paris as 'Parree'.

A couple of foreign languages that are best avoided altogether are management-speak and Hollywood mogul-speak. No one wants to hear anyone talk about getting the heads up to drill down to key deliverables at the end of play nor, indeed, of getting my people to call your people to sunset the project. Say what you mean – it's not hard!

Mastering Foreign Languages

According to a reputable definition of the term 'ladylike', 'a lady should have a working knowledge of at least one foreign language'. It's unfortunate if you have no skills at all in this area, but take heart. Nobody said it had to be one of the conventional 'finishing-school' languages, such as French, German, Italian or Spanish. In fact, if you are going to bluff your way through this ladylike requirement, it's best to choose something pretty obscure, practise a few key phrases and work up a story to match.

What to Choose?

Esperanto will not do. It's just geeky.

Dialects will not do, as they are spoken mainly by peasants and elderly academics.

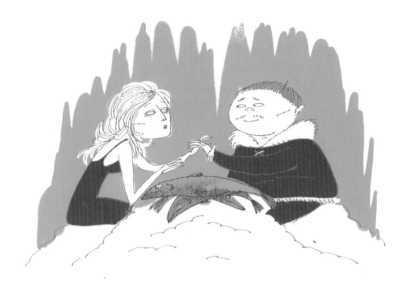

Basque and Celtic languages are too political and might get you into ferocious and unsustainable arguments with a bunch of wild-eyed fanatics.

Greenlandic is an interesting choice: it's sufficiently obscure and could be explained by a thrilling gap-year experience, an absent, explorer father, or an exotic Inuit lover ... although that will bring the small problem of lying about your life (see page 62).

Some useful Greenlandic phrases are:

My hovercraft is full of eels: *Umiat-siaasara pullatt-agaq nimer-ussanik ulikk-aarpoq.*

Would you like to dance with me?: *Qite-qatiger-usuppingaa?*

I love you: *Asavakkit.*

Another approach …

… is to learn one useful phrase in a variety of useless languages:

'This gentleman will pay for everything':

Chinese (Hakka): *Di jak namzai woi wan.*

Croatian: *Ovaj e gospodin sve platiti.*

Icelandic: *Þessi maður mun borga allt saman.*

Zulu: *Umnumzana uzokhokha konke.*

'Call the police!':

Albanian: *Thirrni policinë!*

Latin: *Denuntiatores vocate!*

Somalian: *Booliiska soo wac!*

Welsh: *Galwch yr Heddlu!*

Lunch, Dinner, Supper???

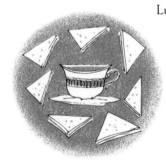

Lunch is the meal we eat at midday. In the evening we eat dinner or supper, depending on the formality of the occasion, and around 4 o'clock we might have tea with a crustless cucumber sandwich and a nice slice of Madeira cake.

Toilets, Dentures And Lounge Rooms

Never use a twirly middle-class euphemism where a nice plain, posh, Anglo-Saxon word will do.

We say	We do not say
Loo or lavatory	Toilet
Scent	Perfume
False teeth	Dentures
Rich	Wealthy
Dead	Passed on
Mad	Mental
Sick	Ill
Graveyard	Cemetery
What?	Pardon?
How do you do?	Pleased to meet you
Dinner jacket	Dress suit
Bike or bicycle	Cycle
House	Home
Sofa	Settee or couch
Sitting room	Lounge or front room
Writing-paper	Notepaper
Good health!	Cheers!
Jam	Preserve
Pudding	Sweet
Vegetables	Greens
Napkin	Serviette
A glass of wine/sherry	A wine/sherry

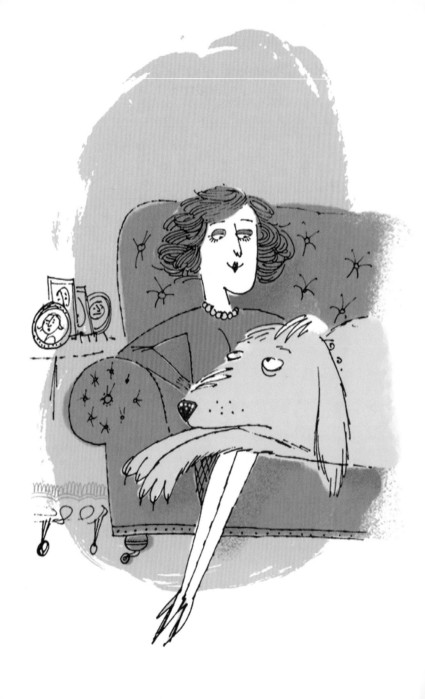

Chapter 4

The Ladylike Lifestyle

———•———

Darling,
when things go wrong in life,
you lift your chin,
put on a ravishing smile,
mix yourself a little cocktail ...

Sophie Kinsella (b. 1969),
best-selling writer of chick-lit.

Jobs For Ladies

A lady is eminently employable, sometimes for her personal merit, sometimes for her connections and address book, but always for her social know-how, impeccable manners and accent.

Art galleries of the more conservative kind (selling muddy landscapes and portraits of horses in gilt frames) are reliable employers of ladies. An attractive girl sporting a velvet Alice band, who sounds as if she might be related to a duke, can instil confidence in nervous buyers even if she doesn't know a Cornetto from a Canaletto.

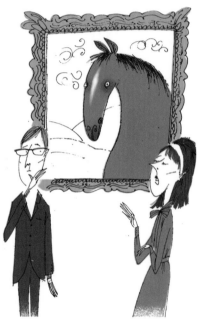

Magazines and newspapers
A novelty column from a girl with connections? Jolly good wheeze, until the ghost writer suffers a sense-of-humour failure.

PR is promising, because employers in this field like ladies with extensive contacts, and ringing round old school chums to persuade them to pop into the latest pop-up restaurant or wear a certain designer's dress to an awards ceremony isn't too taxing.

Party planning is a good choice as the lady is bound to have been to a fabulous number of fabulous parties and be bursting with fabulous ideas.

Interior design is another brilliant choice for the lady. Having been brought up surrounded by beautiful things (or things that were once beautiful and are now faded to a perfect state of stately-home shabby), she has a head start in the taste department.

The way people get their living determines their social outlook.

Karl Marx (1818–1883),
revolutionary socialist and philosopher.

The Real World of Work

Whatever your job, it pays to take a ladylike attitude to your work. This is a cut-throat world, but blatant, naked ambition is very unladylike, and all the effort you have to put in to climb to the top could interfere with long weekends shooting or skiing, shopping and going on safari. So be subtle.

Dress Ambitiously

That means being smart and not distractingly sexy – unless you are a pole dancer, of course. You should be smart in context, though, so if the workplace dress code is jeans and T-shirts, yours are designer jeans and the coolest of T-shirts and shoes. If suits are the code, yours are beautifully well cut and fit fabulously.

Be Smart About Office Politics

Find out who is important and who is not. There's no point in making alliances with people who are on their way out, or with little Hitlers in charge of the stationery supplies. Always be supportive of fellow workers, or at least appear to be. If you are more Machiavelli than Pollyanna, you can tell tales, spread

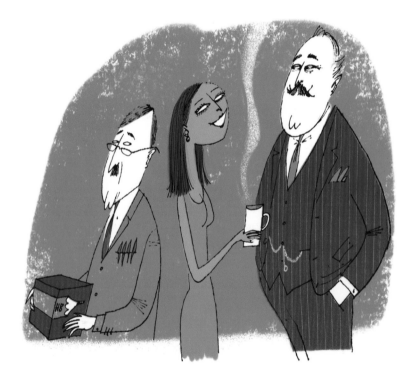

There's no point in making alliances with people
who are on their way out or little Hitlers
in charge of the stationery supplies.

rumours of excessive drinking, talk constantly behind people's backs, store up evidence of misdemeanours and produce damning dossiers with a timely flourish, but be prepared for people to hate you. It's a universal truth that people who are hideous to fellow workers on their way up will regret it mightily in years to come when their career path is strewn with ex-colleagues with very long memories.

Be Professional

Do your job properly and don't leave others to mop up after you. Arrive at work on time and without a hangover, and don't leave early. Aim to get ahead on merit, and do what you can to make sure your merit shines through. Be wary of the 'reply all' button. Be helpful and kind to junior colleagues and never demean anyone in public. Don't spend office time gossiping on the phone to your mother/lover/best friend, or trawling online auctions for second-hand tiaras or copies of *Who's Who*. Don't leave evidence on the office computer network that you may regret (your profile on findmeaposhrichsinglemale.com, for instance).

Be Nice

Share cake. Buy drinks after work on Friday. What goes around comes around.

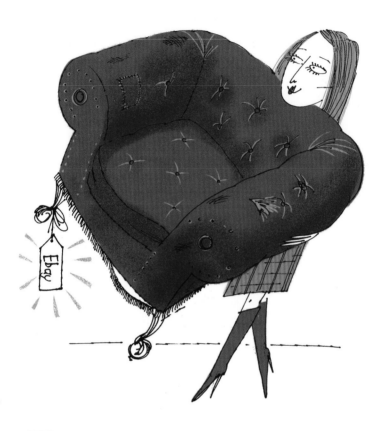

What Your Home Says About You

The IKEA ambiance suggests that you have started with absolutely nothing and have had to buy all your own furniture, which is not ladylike at all. You have to have inherited stuff, or at least own pieces that look inherited, which you then blend cleverly with your mass-market finds in a thoroughly ladylike way.

Floors

Flagstones and proper wooden floorboards are always a good thing. If floorboards are inconsistent or dull, then painting them is a ladylike option. Flooring materials made of one thing and pretending to be another are generally not good, but as always there are some terrific exceptions. Avoid laminated chipboard pretending to be oak, or cheap vinyl patterned with wood grain, for example; but say yes to porcelain tiles that look like polished concrete, and classy pebble-effect vinyl tiles (these are only classy in the bathroom, however).

Ladies will have grown up around fabulous rugs and dense, velvety carpeting specially made for the drawing room 200 years ago by specialist weavers in Bruges. Cheap carpet is most definitely a bad look, so no shag pile, no garish patterns and no 'interesting' colours, please. The best option, which looks both ladylike and cool, is a base of coir matting and a sprinkling of slightly worn oriental rugs. One wonderful lady to whom I am related, when faced with a hideous patterned carpet in a rented home, ripped it up, turned it over, and lived happily for a couple of years with the plain jute backing. A practical decision like this can be considered an über-classy move.

Walls

Heritage paint colours get a big thumbs up, and wallpaper is making a comeback. But there's wallpaper and wallpaper, and, in general, ladies don't do violently edgy. So choose something muted, discreet, faded – maybe a couple of rolls of vintage wallpaper deployed in an alcove. That's the look to aim for.

Curtains

Delicate panels of cheap muslin floating on wires are a bit IKEA, frankly. Heavy velvet, silk damask, swags, tails, pelmets, tie-backs and passementerie,* on the other hand, are good stately-home indicators, but they give out a distinctly middle-aged vibe, and today's lady must be in touch. Chintz goes in and out of style, but as 'good' chintz has an impeccable pedigree, a touch of 'inherited' vintage fabric from Great-aunt eBay could be the way to go – dated and faded, but please, not too ripped. Also ladylike are curtains made from extra-wide heavy-duty artist's canvas, or vintage embroidered French linen sheets, lined and interlined to make them swishy and heavy. These are options with romance and history on their side, an element that is sadly lacking from the instant flat-pack home.

Bedrooms

Is there room for the four-poster bed? The bed drapery will need to be a bit tattered and worn to have any credibility, and you'll definitely need a new mattress. A good, classy alternative is a vintage bed in the French Empire style that shows off a lot of gleaming mahogany and elegant curves. Divans and padded headboards belong in cheap hotels, not in classy boudoirs. Bedlinen should have a high thread count (to show that you're used to luxury), preferably be white and must be clean.

----

* This is a good word to bandy about in ladylike decorating circles. It means elaborate trimmings and edgings made of braid, silken fringes and gold or silver cord.

An antique blanket box at the end of the bed is a good touch, but it would be better to throw stuff on the floor than to stoop to a shiny new flat-packed pine model.

It is possible to economise on nightstands, dressers (chests of drawers) and wardrobes, by making them inconspicuous and blend (decoratively speaking) into the walls. Unnecessary extra pillows or cushions piled on the bed are showy, impractical and therefore not ladylike. A teddy bear is fine, but only if you are young and single and the bear has been loved to raggedy bits and has a Steiff* button in his ear.

Sitting Rooms

You will need sofas that a large dog would find comfortable, an armchair to sit in yourself, a low table to display lovely hard-cover books on art, architecture, dogs and gardens, and a magazine rack holding copies of *Town & Country*, *The Lady*, *Tatler* or *Filthy Rich in The Hamptons Monthly*. It's absolutely necessary to have classy furniture in a sitting room, so haunt auction rooms for family heirlooms in the form of small, affordable antiques such as little writing desks, occasional tables, even footstools. Cover every surface with silver-framed black-and-white photographs of yourself and your family (or someone else's if yours don't measure up), interspersed with shiny trinkets – silver snuff-boxes, for instance. Now you have set the scene, think about lighting. Standard lamps and antique table lamps with impressive handmade silk shades are bulky, but ooze good breeding; directional spotlights might upset the dog.

....

* Steiff is the maker of the classiest possible toy bears.

Cover every flat surface with silver-framed black-and-white photographs of yourself and your family (or someone else's if yours don't measure up).

A well-bred sitting room has non-controversial pictures on the walls and a gilt-framed mirror over a mantelpiece dotted with interesting invitations. You can have a lot of fun faking invitations and finding battered picture frames that need only a bit of glue and gilt paint to live again. If you can't find enough inoffensive muddy landscapes to fill your frames, don't bother, because they probably look better empty on the wall, and there's always scope for an eccentric family bankruptcy story to explain how this situation came about. Never, ever be tempted to hang large family group photographs printed on fake canvas.

Bathrooms

A bathroom obviously needs to be clean. It ought also to smell pleasant because it is well-ventilated and someone has thoughtfully provided a small bowl of home-made pot-pourri or a bunch of sweet-smelling flowers, rather than having an atmosphere tainted with chemical air-fresheners or those blocks of napalm that turn the lavatory water bluer with every flush. As for the equipment, there should be nothing too shiny and new that relies on unseen technology and may confuse elderly relatives. The lavatory should have a proper flush mechanism, not a discreet chrome button masquerading as a dimmer switch. The shower should be powerful and the bath-tub, made of proper old-school enamel-coated steel or cast iron (not fibreglass or acrylic), should be generous and quick to fill.

The downstairs loo is the place for awards, degree certificates, school photographs, cartoons and clipped-out newspaper stories about oneself. That way every visitor is sure to see them and be suitably impressed, but they will also think 'How modest and self-effacing of her to keep her Oscar statuette in the loo! Bless!'

A bathroom needs to be clean and contain flowers and a small bowl of pot-pourri, rather than having an atmosphere tainted with chemical air-fresheners.

Kitchens

Here, it's got to be the country look: battered pine, slate, a deep butler's sink, brand-new old-fashioned brass taps (faucets) with porcelain inserts, an Aga if there's room for one, and open shelves piled with pretty porcelain plates either passed down from mother or collected over the years at vintage fairs. Even the young single lady goes for a version of this look because it's what she grew up with, and luckily IKEA can oblige as far as the units go, helping you to recreate the childhood idyll. The battered pine kitchen table, however, must be a unique find, bringing back memories of cook in her floury apron, working in the scullery rolling out dough and pastry, the muscular figure of the chauffeur leaning casually against the door jamb, dangling the keys to the vintage Hispano-Suiza motor car, framed by views of the dappled sunlit kitchen garden beyond …

Entertaining at Home

As a hostess, the lady has obligations, and thinking about the right mix of guests is perhaps the most important. It is the job of the hostess to make sure that everyone knows what to expect from the evening, and that the guests are comfortable and relaxed, all have drinks in their hands and have all been introduced. It is also her duty to remember that she's invited people and to be ready to receive them. You may think this is stating the obvious, but I know of guests who turned up for dinner to find a startled hostess in her dressing gown having just jumped out of a relaxing bath in preparation for an early night. Try talking your way out of that one. It wasn't easy.

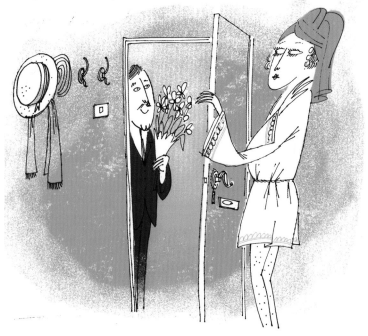

Drinks Parties

Do mention when inviting your guests when you expect them to go home. Make it quite plain whether there will be food or just the odd olive, so they know if they have to plan to eat somewhere else. Unless you have employed half a dozen bar staff, don't attempt to serve too many different kinds of drink. Cocktail parties are a lovely idea, but they do require an awful lot of messing around with measures, different shapes of glass, twists of lemon, swizzle-sticks, shakers and syrups.

If you want to steer away from the usual red, pink, white or beer routine, and are unaccountably short of staff, how about a do-it-yourself gin-and-tonic party? (See page 50 for how to make the perfect G&T.) You provide several flavoured gins, a bucket of ice with tongs, a big icy tub full of tonic-water bottles, plenty of bottle-openers and wedges of lime and lemon, and get people making and mixing their own.

Drinks-party food needs to be bite-size, easy to handle, tasty and plentiful so people can drink without getting too drunk. It's easier to buy in than to slave away making your own mini crayfish tartlets and amusing goujons, because giving parties should be fun and the hostess should be at the beck and call of her guests, not the timer on her oven.

Fruity Gin

- 1 x 70 cl (1¼ pint) bottle bottle gin or vodka (doesn't have to be an expensive brand, but a good one nevertheless, and one with more than 40 per cent alcohol)
- A generous handful of soft fruit, such as raspberries, blackberries, strawberries or blueberries
- Large, clean 1-litre (2-pint) Kilner or Mason jar
- Unbleached coffee filter paper and a funnel

Step one: Put the fruit in the Kilner jar, pour in the gin and seal the jar. Keep in a cool place, gently rocking the jar from side to side every day. Too vigorous a shake will break up the berries and you'll get little filaments floating in your pristine gin. It should be ready to decant in about four days.

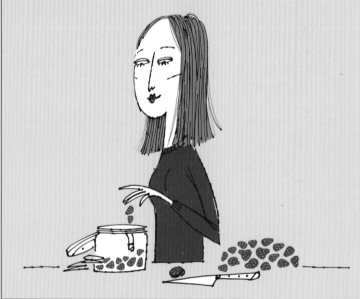

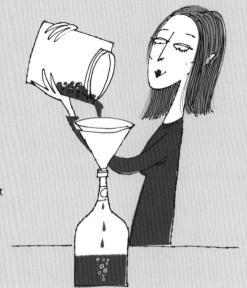

Step two: Decant the flavoured gin into the original bottle using a funnel lined with the filter paper. Discard the fruit.

Step three: Design a label. Party on.

Other flavourings that work well using the same method and the same amount of gin:

Cucumber gin One large cucumber, peeled and all seeds removed, flesh cut into chunks, with a twist of lemon zest.

Ginger gin 300 g (10 oz) piece of fresh, juicy ginger, peeled and cut into chunks.

Earl Grey tea gin Four top-quality Earl Grey teabags (this infusion takes only four hours).

Dinner Parties

These can be either the best way to spend an evening or the worst. If you're organised and in charge, and you know your friends will get on with one another, nothing much can go wrong. If you can't cook, buy in, discard the packaging and serve beautifully – or roast a couple of chickens for an hour, slathered in butter, salt and pepper, with two lemons stuck inside each one.

Laying The Table

The act of calmly preparing the scene for your party can be very soothing, so leave yourself enough time to enjoy the moment. Smooth out a clean tablecloth, sort out plates for starters and main dishes, place napkins and cutlery (flatware) just so, with side plates to the left. Water glasses go to the right of wine glasses. Keep any flowers low and unobtrusive. Lighting should be soft and flattering, with candles or oil lamps primed and ready. Have a vague idea of where you will seat people, but keep it flexible. You should separate couples, alternate men and women within reason, and seat people with similar interests together, placing yourself nearest to the kitchen.

Sascha had decided she liked cooking. Unfortunately, cooking didn't like her back.

Nalini Singh,
Branded by Fire (2009)

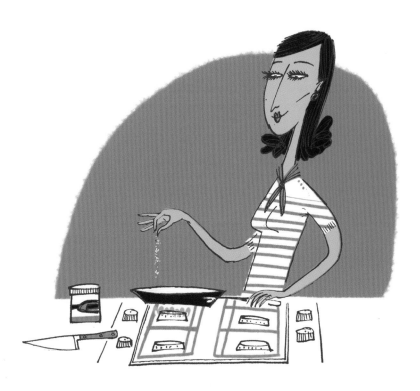

Cooking Like a Lady

Not everyone is interested in cooking, or is any good at it, but it is my theory that a lady should be able to do a few things exceptionally well. Perfecting a dinner-party dish or two and being able to serve up a decent breakfast are necessary life skills.

No one is born a great cook, one learns by doing.

Julia Child,
My Life in France (2006)

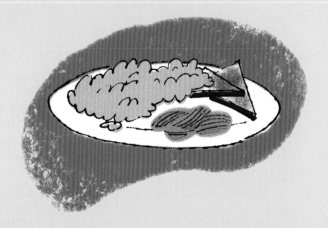

A Ladylike Breakfast

Every lady should be famous for a breakfast dish. The timing for a proper full English breakfast consisting of bacon and eggs is full of pitfalls, and anyway the idea of frying is too greasy to be ladylike. Practise this recipe for scrambled egg with smoked salmon: by cooking some of the salmon and leaving the rest raw, you get two different flavours and textures. It's the perfect classy breakfast.

For two people

- 4 fresh eggs
- 1 tablespoon crème fraîche
- salt and pepper
- handful of fresh parsley
- 4 slices smoked salmon
- two slices wholemeal bread
- butter

Prepare the egg mixture

Break the eggs into a mixing bowl, whisk them up and add the crème fraîche and a little salt and pepper. Chop the parsley and set aside.

Prepare the smoked salmon and start the toast

Cut two of the slices of salmon into strips and then slice across the strips making pieces approximately 5 cm (2 in.) long. Start toasting the bread.

Cook the eggs

Melt the butter in a non-stick pan. Stir the chopped salmon into the eggs. When the butter foams, add the egg mixture to the pan and keep stirring, pulling the set egg off the bottom of the pan until all the egg has formed into soft curds.

Serve

Take the pan off the heat, and add a little more butter. Quickly butter the toast, arrange a slice of smoked salmon to one side and then divide the cooked egg between the two slices of toast. Grind black pepper over the egg and salmon, decorate with parsley and eat immediately.

One should not attend even the end of the world without a good breakfast.

Robert A. Heinlein,
Friday (1982)

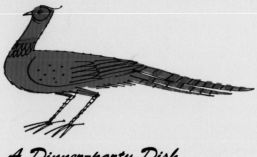

A Dinner-party Dish

There's nothing too gourmet here – no seared scallops, no *jus* of any kind, and no boned quails *en papillote*. This is a down-to-earth but ladylike pheasant casserole, made with ingredients culled from the estate with total disregard to waste. After all, during the pheasant season these birds are cheaper than chips.

For four people

- 2 pheasants or, as we say up at the big house, a brace of pheasants
- bunch of celery, washed
- 1 onion, peeled
- 1 cooking apple, cored
- butter and oil for frying
- 1 tablespoon plain flour
- salt and pepper
- 1 teaspoon juniper berries
- strip of orange zest
- 600 ml (1 pint) decent cider
- 2 tablespoons drunken sultanas or raisins (steeped in cheap brandy – a brilliant pick-me-up for all kinds of stews, casseroles and cooks)
- 1 tablespoon crème fraiche (maybe more)

Prepare the pheasants

It's a good idea to practise this on a few birds until you get the hang of it. Put each pheasant breast up on a chopping board, put the heel of your hand over the breast bone and push down, breaking bones as you go. Now wiggle the legs around to loosen them and slice them off with a sharp knife, aiming to cut them from the carcass at the joint. Arming yourself now with a decent pair of poultry shears, snip out the entire backbone and any ribs you can easily get at, then cut through the breastbone (you should have broken the wishbone, so it's not as hard to do this as it sounds). Each pheasant should now be in four pieces – two legs and two breasts. Trim away anything unsightly.

Prepare the vegetables

Chop the celery, onion and apple (don't bother to peel the apple).

Sear the pheasants

Put the butter and oil into a large, heavy casserole dish. While it heats up, dredge the pheasant pieces in flour, salt and pepper. Give them a shake to get rid of any excess flour, and pop them into the pan. Brown them well on all sides, without letting the flour burn, then fish them out and keep to one side.

Soften the vegetables

Pile the vegetables into the pan and stir until they begin to go soft. Make sure the heat is not too high as you want to soften the vegetables rather than brown them. Add the juniper berries, any excess flour and the orange zest.

Throw everything in together

Now put back the pheasant pieces, stir a bit, and add the cider and drunken raisins. Put the lid on slightly askew, turn the heat down to a simmer and let it cook for about an hour, checking the meat now and then – undercooked pheasant is tough and unpleasant, but overcooked it is flabby and tasteless. For the last ten minutes, take off the lid to help the cider sauce to thicken and reduce. Finally, stir in the crème fraîche, heat through and serve from the pot. Mind the lead shot.

 Tip: Get the footman to mash the potatoes for you.

A Late-night Snack

Here's how to make a divinely simple steak sandwich, very popular for those late-night munchies.

For one person

- 1 rump steak about 1 cm (½ in.) thick (that's quite thin)
- salt and pepper
- drizzle of oil
- 2 thick slices of crusty white bread
- good-quality salted butter
- salad leaves

Cook the steak

Heat a griddle pan over a high flame until it begins to smoke. While you are waiting, season the steak with salt and pepper and

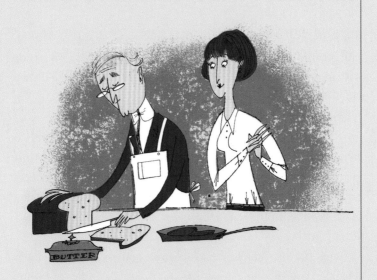

massage a little oil into it. Just when you think the pan is going to explode, throw in the steak and cook for just over a minute on each side.

Assemble the sandwich

Butter the bread. Put the salad leaves on one piece, and balance the smokin' steak on top. Slap on the top slice and turn the sandwich over so the cooking juices run into the salad leaves. Bliss. You may want to gain some marks for presentation by cutting the sandwich in half and serving it on a plate with a couple of slices of tomato and a sprinkling of fresh parsley.

Alternatively, get the butler to make it for you.

Ladylike Pleasures And Passions

Shopping is good (for clothes, not groceries). Planning parties, philanthropy, playing the piano, painting, drawing and gardening with proper gloves and a big shady hat, are all well-established ladylike hobbies.

Cooking is a very respectable pleasure these days, but avoid anything too niche, such as exclusively baking cupcakes, which rather smacks of obsession. Crafty things, such as scrapbooking, creating handmade paper from rags and sticking cut-out images on to random surfaces (découpage, they call it), are a bit middle-class, frankly. Knitting is enjoying a ladylike revival, but cross-stitch, crochet and needlepoint are still naff.

Travel is a top passion, but avoid cruises unless they are to polar regions. Trekking up mountains on horseback and following pilgrimage paths in the footsteps of saints have an eccentric ladylike authenticity that is hard to beat.

Exercise classes and running are good; body-building is beyond bad. Boot-camp activities are just a bit too 'keen'. Ladies should not get too hot and sweaty.

Singing in a choir hits all the right buttons. In fact, making music of any kind is most commendable – even learning to play the recorder properly is an achievement not to be denigrated.

Bridge, backgammon, poker and Scrabble get a thumbs up; dominoes and Trivial Pursuit a thumbs down. Chess is obviously an eminently suitable game, but only if you're good at it.

Reading is on everybody's CV as a hobby, but it depends what you read, of course. Well-written thrillers are quite the thing at the moment; chick-lit beach reads are just about okay as long as you have the chutzpah to chuck them in the sea with a sigh of shame the moment you finish. Literary fiction is rewarding and displays impeccable taste. It is never necessary to join a book club.

Ballet and opera go with the territory as strawberries go with cream. Theatre- and movie-going are culturally sound, but beware of the coach-party level of theatrical experience. If you're going to be a film buff, be sure to pick a genre, actor or director and immerse yourself. Displaying an eccentric passion for the films of the French Nouvelle Vague, for instance, will do wonders for your ladylike credentials.

Being Sporty

Ladies have to know how to ride a horse, ski, sail and play tennis. Although you don't have to be brilliant at all these, it is important to know the rules and how to be an amenable and pleasant playmate, which means not trying to win all the time.

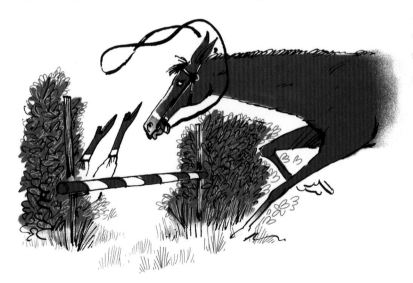

Golf and fly-fishing are added extras. Team games such as field hockey, lacrosse and netball are best abandoned after leaving school because they mean being keen, joining a club and training seriously, all of which could get in the way of the lifestyle.

Getting The Outfit Right

This is almost more important than being able to play the game. The perils of 'all the gear but no idea' have already been touched on (see page 26). Ladies will know instinctively which item of clothing or piece of equipment is really important for getting the message of impeccable breeding across in one go. Bear in mind that anything too new looks as if you had to rush out and buy it, which is frankly déclassé and could have you mistaken for a nouveau-riche Russian. This applies particularly to ski outfits. Ladies should have all the 'right' stuff piled up in the tack room or packed away in trunks. For riding, boots have to be classy, but it doesn't matter if they're muddy and scuffed and you are wearing jeans. Good deck shoes will take you sailing just about anywhere, but you will also need the right kind of waterproofs. Tennis outfits should be white – Wimbledon rules apply here – and rackets should be well used. Sporting clothing can be old and even a bit frayed, but it should never, ever have been cheap to buy in the first place.

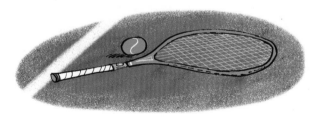

Nothing is perfect. Life is messy. Relationships are complex. Outcomes are uncertain. People are irrational.

Hugh Mackay (b. 1938),
Australian psychologist and social researcher.

The Dark Side

Ladies should obviously keep their eyes and hearts on nabbing a prize catch, but living life as if you're Little Miss Manners all the time is dull, and being dull and predictable is social death. The fact is that everyone warms to a lady with edge, and eccentricity is as highly prized a ladylike quality as impeccable *savoir faire*. Ideally, of course, the two should go together, and the lady, when adding to her street cred by getting down with unsuitably tattooed drug dealers, will not let her standards slip. She will always remember to say please and thank you, pass the salt without being asked twice, and never refer to the toilet (it's a lavatory).

Everyone needs a bit of excitement and a stash of tales of a misspent youth with which to give complexes to the children and impress the grandchildren. When safely married off to Peregrine Smug-Moneybags, what fun it is for a lady to hold forth with stories of a life led well away from the charmed, safe circle of posh – a string of dangerous dalliances with rappers, cage fighters, bouncers, boxers and that creepy guy from Technical Support. However – and perhaps this is easier said than done – it's not a good idea to get so far in that you can't get out.

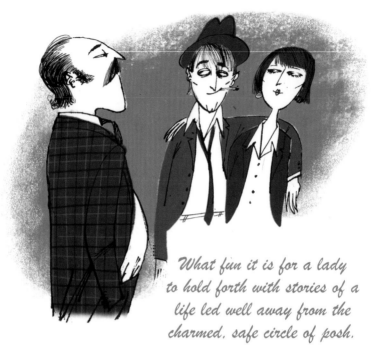

What fun it is for a lady to hold forth with stories of a life led well away from the charmed, safe circle of posh.

Drugs

Lords and ladies, dukes and duchesses, ladies and gentlemen, boys and girls – they can all get as out of it as anyone else. And yes, it seems to be frightfully good fun, and one's drug dealer might be the wittiest, kindest, loveliest human being on the planet, and the inside of your own brain the only place you ever want to visit, but there comes a time (before too much damage has been done, it is to be hoped) when the lady must summon up the necessary backbone to wipe her nose clean, lose the supplier's phone number, get to grips with reality and take up gardening.

Relationships

The lady will always be charming, interested, polite and kind to everyone whether duchess or dinner lady – and she'll somehow manage that without being creepy or patronising. It's a difficult balance to get right, and it's called class.

In affairs of the heart, it doesn't do to be too keen too soon. Everyone knows that. But that does not mean you should be a polite, hopeful little face in the background waiting for an approach. Be bold in your signals of interest; just don't let your opening gambit be the choice of wedding venues.

If relationships are going to work, they will develop at a natural pace. Share stuff about yourself and expect the same in return. Enjoy yourself and make yourself a fun and attractive person to be around. If you fall in love this will all come naturally and the tiresome he-said/she-said, will-he/won't-he dramas will get relegated to the back burner where they belong.

Keep your counsel – that's a good piece of advice. Don't blabber or witter or twitter to the world at large about a new person in your life; it's never a good idea to keep up a running commentary on a fledgling relationship. It's not only deeply unladylike, with overtones of the emotional incontinence displayed by orange-skinned Z-listers, but it could also turn out to be humiliating, hurtful and embarrassing.

It's Over!

If it's been short-lived, and he ends it, the lady will take the message on board and walk away with her head held high. Do not go back for more. If a long-term affair hits the buffers, go and cry somewhere private and don't even think about attempting emotional blackmail. If you still feel the hurt can be excised only in a drastic way, plot a slow and delicious revenge (see page 120).

If you end it, be kind and reasonable and don't go into too much detail about why and what's wrong with him, as that is tacky. Just go, leaving a whiff of scent and a superior air of mystery. Don't let someone down by txt msg – a goodbye is at least worth a phone call. If you are serious about it being over, don't let even a glimmer of hope linger, or he'll pester you and you'll be wrung out with unnecessary guilt.

Don't flirt with his friends. Don't sleep with his friends, unless of course you want to be frozen out of the circle and consigned to the outer darkness. If he tries the same trick on your friends, ditch him immediately – only misery awaits. Love is arbitrary, but if you sense a pattern of control freakery and/or humiliating put-downs, pack your heart away safely along with your toothbrush and get out. And it should go without saying that you must never stay for one moment with a man, however charming and well-bred on the surface, who hits you or threatens to do so. To stay is to let down the whole of womankind.

I like my relationships like I like my eggs. Over easy.

Jarod Kintz,
It Occurred to Me (2010)

One-night Stands

These are risky, not only for your reputation, but also for your health and safety. If you feel it's okay, then try to steer the event so that it is at your place, not his. That way you remain in charge and avoid the walk of shame (going home in last night's clothes). Don't get too involved by sharing hopes and dreams or personal information, otherwise what could be a mutually beneficial sex-without-strings thing risks turning into a messy liaison with expectations and guilt and all the rest of the baggage you were presumably hoping to avoid. You could always pretend to be someone else.

Have a plausible excuse ready for the morning after. The idea of your mother visiting from out of town should get him moving pretty quickly. Give him some breakfast, and be charming even if you have a monster hangover. You don't want to compound any hint of shame you may be experiencing by being nasty, dismissive and unladylike, as the whole idea was to enjoy the experience for what it was.

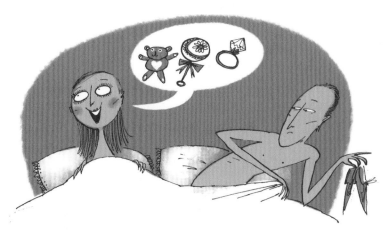

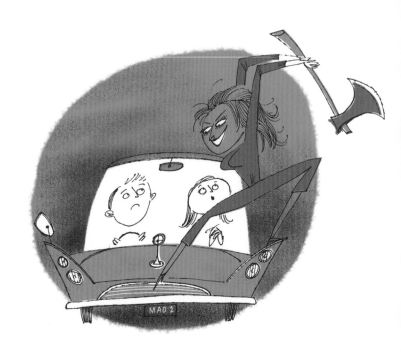

Ladylike Ways
to Mete Out Revenge

Looking absolutely stunning at an event your ex is bound to hear about or attend will certainly make you feel better about yourself, and it is a classy move. Whether looking gorgeous will bring him to heel is questionable, as people don't normally fall out of love with people because of the way they look, but because of the way they are. No one is going to forget the Revenge Dress worn by Princess Diana on the day her prince confessed to adultery with a homely woman of a certain age, but – despite making her point – she didn't get him back.

Gorgeous hair is the best revenge.

Ivana Trump (b. 1949),
celebrity with a bouffant.

Neuroscientists tell us that the bit of our brain known as the dorsal striatum, which lights up at the prospect of reward, also goes into overdrive at the thought of revenge. So there you have it: scientific proof that revenge is sweet. Here are some interesting tales of women who have given their dorsal striatum free rein.

His Things!

There are several instances of wronged women making bonfires of a cheating ex's clothes, gathering the ashes and delivering the urn to the door; putting the house up for sale; and selling all his stuff on eBay. The poster girl for revenge on possessions has to be Lady Sarah Graham-Moon, who was in the midst of what she thought was a civilised, living-under-the-same-roof divorce from her minor aristocrat husband when he compounded his sins by having an affair with a neighbour. So she let rip: she poured gallons of white paint over his beloved Jaguar car, distributed the contents of his vintage wine collection around the village and cut up all his bespoke suits. Way to go, girl!

His Penis!

This is perhaps not the most ladylike of revenge scenarios, but boy, was it effective. In 1993 Lorena Bobbitt, a wronged and abused wife from Virginia, finally snapped: during the night, after

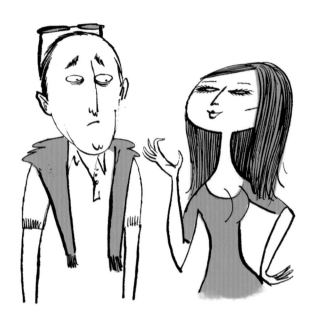

her husband, John Wayne Bobbitt, had allegedly attempted to rape her, she sliced off his penis with a carving knife. She then jumped into the car, drove around for a bit and threw his manhood out of the window.

What happened next? There was a court hearing, but neither was charged with a crime. His penis was reattached, and he cashed in on the notoriety and founded an unsuccessful band called The Severed Parts. She started an organisation to help victims of domestic abuse and marital rape. The couple divorced.

If you are hestitant about the prospect of mutilating your partner's genitals, you can feel proud that you are a well-balanced, rational lady. However, if the urge to verbally hit a gentleman who has wronged you where it hurts, a well-timed quip questioning the size of his manhood should do the trick.

His Liberty! His Reputation! His Life!

In the early years of the twentieth century, Dr Hawley Harvey Crippen, a not very successful homeopathic doctor, was living in London with his wife, Cora, an American concert singer. Unfortunately, it wasn't a happy marriage: Mrs Crippen had an affair with one of their lodgers, and Dr Crippen took up with a young typist called Ethel. Miffed, Cora announced that she was leaving for America, along with the couple's money, which was mostly hers. Shortly afterwards, she went missing and was never seen again.

Dr Crippen told friends and relatives that she'd fallen ill and died after arriving in Los Angeles. He then sold his wife's jewellery collection, gave his landlord notice and planned to set sail with Ethel to start a new life in the United States. Mrs Crippen's friends suspected foul play and promptly alerted the police. Dr Crippen's home was investigated and a body was found in the cellar. He was convicted of his wife's murder and hanged in 1910. In 2007, forensic examination proved that the remains hadn't been those of Cora after all; in fact, they had belonged to a man.

So what was the story? Did Cora stage-manage the whole thing? Did she deliberately lie low when she realised they'd found a body in the cellar? When they hanged her husband, did she throw a cocktail party? Or did Dr Crippen dispose of his wife's remains elsewhere? Who was the body in the cellar? Where did Cora end up?

Put-downs

Practise withering looks in front of the mirror. If withering doesn't cut it, it's time for a poisoned barb – and timing is all-important. Pause until you have the full attention of your audience, pop in your line and try not to look too smug. It would be a shame to waste a good build-up by limping out with a mere playground taunt, so study the masters, learn and adapt. Here are some sample barbs from the best practitioners of the art of the put-down:

When talking about someone with a questionable personality:

It'd be a terrific innovation if you could stretch your mind a little further than the next wisecrack

Katharine Hepburn

A modest little person, with much to be modest about

Winston Churchill

He has no enemies, but is intensely disliked by his friends

Oscar Wilde

I've just learned about his illness. Let's hope it's nothing trivial

Irvin S. Cobb

He had delusions of adequacy

Walter Kerr

— ❦ —

He has all the virtues I dislike and none of the vices I admire

Winston Churchill

— ❦ —

His mother should have thrown him away and kept the stork

Mae West

— ❦ —

I didn't attend the funeral, but I sent a nice letter saying I approved of it

Mark Twain

— ❦ —

He is a self-made man and worships his creator

John Bright

— ❦ —

I have never killed a man, but I have read many obituaries with great pleasure

Clarence Darrow

Exit lines:
I refuse to have a battle of wits with an unarmed opponent

Anonymous

— ❦ —

If you're gonna be two-faced,
at least make one of them pretty
Kayla Morris

— ~ —

You've a body to die for, and a face to protect it
Anonymous

— ~ —

I've had a perfectly wonderful evening, but this wasn't it
Groucho Marx

— ~ —

Talk to me. I could do with the sleep
Anonymous

— ~ —

You could light up the room just by leaving it
Anonymous

— ~ —

The next time you wash your neck, wring it
Anonymous

— ~ —

Don't go away; I want to forget you exactly as you are!
Anonymous

— ~ —

I wish I had known you when you were alive
Leonard Lewis Levison

CODA
A Final Piece of Advice

Some things just have to be shared – especially this, tip number nine for choosing a husband from the deservedly long-forgotten book of lifestyle advice **Light on Dark Corners**: *A Complete Sexual Science and a Guide to Purity and Physical Manhood; Advice to Maiden, Wife and Mother; Love, Courtship and Marriage* by B.G. Jefferis and J.L. Nichols, first published in the United States in 1895:

Do not marry a man with a low, flat head; for, however fascinating, genteel, polite, tender, plausible or winning he may be, you will repent the day of your espousal.

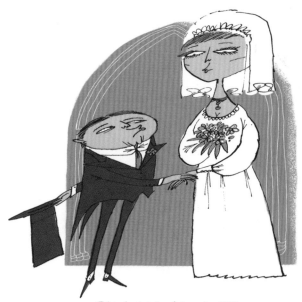

Index

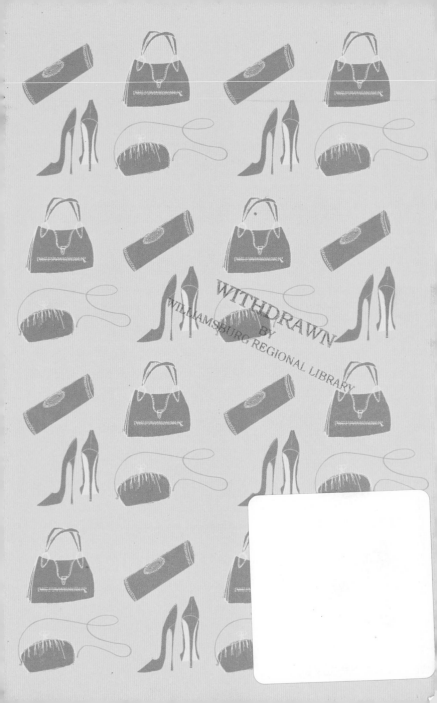